COUPLE'S MASSAGE
H A N D B O O K

Deepen Your Relationship with the
Healing Power of Touch

HELEN HODGSON

Published by: Serve The Goddess

Interior Design: Stefan Merour
Editing: Frank Steele
Illustrator: Vladimir Cebu
Photographer: Jaymie Garner
Cover Book Designer: Jeannie Shaw

ISBN: 978-0-692-76278-3

FOREWORD

After the honeymoon is over, couples often retreat into old habits and patterns that create distance and disconnection. We can lose the spark and excitement we once had and yearn for a deeper, more passionate connection with our partner. This is when creating a new ritual or practice is vital for the intimacy and longevity of your union. *The Couple's Massage Handbook* is absolutely the best way to deepen your relationship with the healing power of touch.

Helen Hodgson is an advocate for empowering women to practice extreme self-care and self-love by inspiring them to access their inner Goddess through reverence, rejuvenation, relaxation, and the healing power of touch. She and Serve the Goddess have been doing just that for over 15 years.

Imagine sitting at your desk and having hands start to gently rub your neck and shoulders. The warmth of the hands on your back and the increasingly strong circular patterns moving up and down your back inspires you to close your eyes and melt into your chair. *Who is this massage therapist behind me?* you think. It's your partner, who has learned how to use basic massage strokes from *The Couple's Massage Handbook*!

How many times have you wanted a massage and not made time for it? Or maybe you didn't allow yourself the budget for this experience. *The Couple's Massage Handbook i*s not only a way to experience relaxation and rejuvenation in your own body; it is a way to deeply connect with your partner and ignite your relationship.

As you embark on this journey together, you will learn some of the benefits of massage, such as stress relief. Even a single massage can significantly lower heart rate, cortisol, and insulin levels, which help reduce daily stress. Massage can play an important role in relieving respiratory issues and training the body how to relax. Got a headache? Forty-five million Americans suffer from chronic headaches and migraines. Massage helps ease the pressure and pain, which can also reduce the frequency of headaches. Want to fight colds? A massage can strengthen your immune system. These are just a few of the health benefits you will learn about in *The Couple's Massage Handbook*.

How easy is it to learn how to massage? I can tell you from personal experience that Helen makes it very easy to follow her directions, with detailed instruction and pictures. Combined with the love and energy of your very own partner, the resulting touch is magic.

By using *The Couple's Massage Handbook,* you not only create better health for you and your loved one, you also reignite the spark that connects you on a level that only touch can activate. The way to bring more love into the world is to start with how you love yourself and those closest to you. By using this book regularly, you not only energize your own relationship and body, you also infuse love energy into the world to create more peace, joy, and happiness for everyone.

JJ Flizanes
Host of The Fit 2 Love Podcast Show and Author of *Fit 2 Love: How to Get Physically, Emotionally and Spiritually Fit to Attract the Love of Your Life.*
Los Angeles, CA, 2016

DEDICATION

I dedicate this book to my husband Dave.
You are my anchor and the love of my life.

ACKNOWLEDGMENTS

I'd like to express my deepest gratitude to my clients and future clients. You are the motivation behind the creation of this book. I couldn't have done it without you.

A special thank-you to the following people.

Frank Steele, editor, for your expertise and time in polishing the manuscript. Vladimir Cebu, illustrator, for your skills and contribution to the book. Designers Stefan Merour and Jeannie Shaw; you really took this book to another level.

My appreciation to models JJ and Brian. Thank you for your enthusiasm and adaptability during our photo shoot. Your dedication is a testament to your marriage.

Jaymie Garner, photographer, for capturing the beautiful images that brought the strokes to life.

My mentor and coach Mary Lyn Miller for keeping me on track, and for her endless inspiration and insight.

I am thankful for my mastermind groups for keeping me accountable and stretched.

To my wonderful team of massage therapists, aestheticians, and nail technicians who provide massage and spa services to my mobile spa clients at Serve The Goddess. My assistant, Jeannie, for the support running my mobile spa business, especially during this book project.

I am forever in gratitude to my husband for his support and patience.

And to my dear mother, I miss you every day.

Thank you all for making this book possible.

FREE GIFT

THE COUPLE'S MASSAGE CHECKLIST

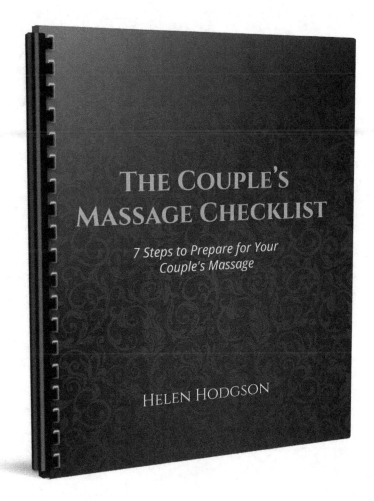

DOWNLOAD HERE:
http://www.servethegoddess.com/couple-massage-checklist

Put the lessons from the handbook into practice by preparing for your first couple's massage. Download your checklist and tool guide now.

CONTENTS

CHAPTER 1:
Back Over Time

WHAT YOU'LL LEARN

❖ The origins of massage for healing purposes
❖ Touch techniques around the world
❖ Cool facts in the history of massage
❖ Where massage is today

Human touch is as old as life itself.

Imagine yourself back in the good old days of the cave dwellers. There's Grud, on his way home from slaying a woolly mammoth, hauling the monstrous creature's carcass. There's Ila, mother to his children, sitting in the glacial cave, just returned from gathering brush and berries from the surrounding wilderness. As darkness begins to fall, Ila turns to Grud and whispers, "Maybe later we do the touch thing?" He grunts back a friendly "Ugh," then turns his attention to carving meat off the mammoth.

OOGA BOOGA! ONE TOUCH IS WORTH A THOUSAND WORDS

After all their offspring are tucked under their furs, with the fire casting a warm glow on them, Grud and Ila lie together and tenderly touch each other's bodies. Grud bites into a wild apple to sweeten his breath, then draws Ila's mouth to him, sharing the sweet morsel of fruit and heightening her olfactory senses. Next, she applies the oil of musk ox to his flesh, softening his rough skin. He lies quietly under the wrap with her, allowing her fingers to penetrate his tired muscles, understanding this to be her signal for romance.

The primal *oohs* and *aahs* from cave men and women enjoying their couple's massages were probably some of the first sounds of pleasure uttered in those early human settlements.

CURSES, BONES, AND TRINKETS: ANCIENT CULTURES OF MASSAGE

As humans evolved, so did their touch techniques. For example, archaeologists have found stone probes in Chinese caves and tombs that were used to soothe aches and pains. Loved ones, it seems, would lay the tools against sore muscles and the soles of the feet, thereby relieving aches and pains throughout the body. Humans were beginning to discover the inner universe of the body, including the sources of their discomforts and even diseases.

Mongolian horsemen were also known to use stones to relax tense muscles. Before going into battle, the warriors would receive a stone massage, during which their fears, believed to be trapped inside of their muscles, would be released. When all the muscles were loose and relaxed, the warriors were ready for battle. So even in ancient times, massage was much more than a physical relaxant—it also helped to heal the body and embolden the spirit.

Soon other early massage techniques began to sprout up around the globe.

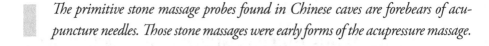

The primitive stone massage probes found in Chinese caves are forebears of acupuncture needles. Those stone massages were early forms of the acupressure massage.

DON'T ASP ME! EGYPT AND CLEOPATRA

Egyptian hieroglyphs, which date from 2500 BCE, are filled with depictions of Egyptians receiving an early form of *reflexology*. Somehow the Egyptians had discovered that tension in any part of the feet reflected stress clusters in corresponding parts of the body. These corresponding parts have appeared in drawings and charts as far back as the building of the Egyptian pyramids. The simple act of giving a foot rub began to take on deeper meaning.

> *Vladimir Bekhterev first referred to the science of reflex therapy as "Reflexology" in 1917.* **Reflexology** *is a therapy in which the feet or hands are pressed to bring relief to corresponding areas of the body.*

No doubt the Egyptian queen Cleopatra knew of massage and used it along with her ravishing beauty to seduce Julius Caesar. It is said that Cleopatra went to great lengths to understand all the sensual desires of a man. She spent her days plying men with wine and women until she seduced her prey, always exceeding his sensual expectations.

And Cleopatra knew that all the senses could be used to invoke the senses. When the black beauty sailed down the Nile to seduce Caesar's rival, Marc Antony, she soaked the sails of her ship in the scent of jasmine to perfume the night air, leaving a trail of seduced admirers. Her barge was lined with the most beautiful of her women, exquisitely attired maidens who also pulled the oars and controlled the sails. On the deck of the barge a massive incense burner was kept aflame with heaps of Kyphi, the richest of Egyptian scented offerings. They mixed oils of cassia, cinnamon, peppermint, pistacia, juniper, acacia, henna, and cypress, then soaked the aromatic mixture in wine and added honey, resins, and myrrh. Can't you just picture the barge floating as if on a cloud of sensual intoxication, mesmerizing all the men she passed by?

> *Cleopatra was known for her beauty, including her beautiful skin. Try one of Cleopatra's milk baths—it is a great remedy for dry, itchy, and nutrient-deficient skin. First take a shower, then prepare a warm bath with 2 cups of whole milk, 2 cups of powdered milk, and 5 to 10 drops of your favorite scented oils. Then lie and soak, relaxing for about 20 minutes. Next, gently dry yourself and apply a moisturizer with vitamin E or natural aloe vera.*

While Cleopatra was relaxing in her bath, musicians played ambient music. Afterward she would have a maiden remove any excess hair, apply henna for eyeliner and specially prepared makeup that enhanced the beauty of her skin and at the same time protected it from the harmful rays of the sun.

Once on board her vessel, so the tale goes, Marc Antony fell prey to Cleopatra's charms. While "holding court" with the lovely queen (I'm being polite here), Marc Antony reportedly reached out and began to massage Cleopatra's manicured toes and oiled feet. I don't believe for a second that he stopped there, but you can fill in the blanks. Poor Marc Antony never stood a chance.

THOSE DECADENT ROMANS!

Asclepiades, a Greek physician, brought massage to Rome. It wasn't long before it was part of the Roman lifestyle. Servants massaged the rich in their homes, while the average Roman went to the public baths for his touch treatment. Massage became the essential treatment for all that ailed the receiver. Those imaginative Romans even believed that massage could replace exercise and the harmful effects of overindulgence in alcohol. If only that were true!

Romans used full-body massage to arouse the senses and nerves, to make the joints limber, and to improve circulation. They rubbed very fine oil all over their bodies to keep the skin supple and young-looking, as well as fragrant.

Galen, a physician to several emperors of the second century CE, including Marcus Aurelius, prescribed massage as a treatment for many disorders. Galen learned about massage from administering to the health needs of the gladiators and from studying the human body. He believed in the importance of moderation in life, and emphasized the use of massage and hydrotherapy (the use of water to treat diseases or injuries) as a positive part of a balanced life of work, pleasure, sex, alcohol, and exercise. History shows Galen's wise advice fell on deaf ears as the decadent lifestyle of the average Roman contributed more to the corruption and decline of the empire than any warring enemy ever did.

Julius Caesar suffered from many nervous disorders, including epilepsy. According to legend, if not for his daily massages—or "pinching," as they called it—Caesar would not have been able to carry on as leader of Rome.

The Romans made massage popular, but it was the Greek men of medicine—such as Asclepiades and Hippocrates—who introduced it to them.

AH SO! ANCIENT CULTURES OF THE FAR EAST

The oldest known book about massage was *The Cong-Fou of Tao-Tse*, written in China in 3000 BCE. In the 1700s, the book was translated into French. In ancient China the most widely used massage of the time was called "Anmo," which literally means "pressing and rubbing." Archaeologists have found massage treatments for illnesses inscribed on bones as far back as the Shang Dynasty in the sixteenth through eleventh centuries BCE.

Around 1400 BCE, the Chinese developed a highly elaborate system that charted the flow of chi (energy) in the body along meridians. Chi travels in the same way neurotransmitters travel along the nerves throughout our body. The difference is that meridians are believed to be paths that convey energy and vital force—a system like our nervous system, but more delicate and less tangible. The Chinese believed (and many still do) that all illnesses are due to imbalances in the flow of chi. Massage is one of the many techniques the Chinese developed to balance the flow of chi. Chinese massage, called acupressure massage, applies pressure to specific points along the meridians to balance the flow of chi.

The Chinese relied on herbs, acupressure massage, and acupuncture treatments (use of needles on those same acupressure points), to create balance, flow, and wellness.

There is an old Chinese story dating back to 5000 BCE about a wife who deeply mourned the death of her husband. As was the custom in that day, the body was prepared for burial and, once it was ready, pallbearers carried the body around the outside of the deceased person's home three times. As the pall-

5

> *bearers made their final trip around the house with the woman's husband, they bumped his foot on a corner. Suddenly the husband revived and sat up!*
>
> *According to the legend, the blow to the foot hit a chi point (which later came to be called Bubbling Spring, also known as Kidney-1) on the sole of the foot. Bumping this point brought the husband out of a deep coma. He survived in good health for another three years, when he died. At the second funeral, the widow implored the pallbearers to be careful not to bump her husband's feet!*

Over time, couple's massage flourished around the world. Imagine, for example, if you could travel back in history to peek into the rooms of a medieval castle. You might see, hear, or smell some wild things behind the velvet drapes. Thinking back to days of chain mail, helmets, armor that dragged you down the stairs from the sheer weight of the suits, conjures up a nonsensual life. Perhaps, though, behind the massive castle walls, inside some rounded turret, a maiden rub-a-dub-dubbed her princely boyfriend, or a guard stole midnight kisses from his sweetheart while caressing the nape of her quivering neck.

GOING SWEDISH: THE STORY OF PETER LING

Massage started getting some mainstream attention in the West in the late 1700s and early 1800s thanks to a gymnastics instructor from Sweden. Professor Peter Ling, who suffered severe rheumatism, read a French translation of *The Cong-Fou of Tao-Tse*, the ancient Chinese text describing massage. Mr. Ling combined his knowledge of physiology, gymnastics, and experiments with the Chinese massage techniques to cure his rheumatism. He called his massage and exercise therapies the Swedish movement system.

Today the Swedish movement system has evolved into Swedish massage. Ling's technique was eventually endorsed by the Swedish government, which conferred respectability on it. A successor of Mr. Ling, Dr. Johann Mezger, was influential in bringing massage to mainstream physicians as a scientific treatment of pain and disease. The practice became popular in Britain around 1814.

The widely practiced technique includes the following movements:

- ❖ **Effleurage.** These are long, gliding, fluid strokes that are sure to make your honey purr.
- ❖ **Petrissage.** Pick up the muscles and squeeze, roll, or wring them like kneading dough.
- ❖ **Friction or circular rubbing.** The skin will flush, creating heat.
- ❖ **Tapotement or Percussion.** Practice your drumming skills here with tapping, cupping, and clapping.
- ❖ **Vibration or Shaking.** A trembling movement that actually feels pretty good.

MAINSTREAMING TOUCH: FROM EUROPE TO THE UNITED STATES

By 1860 Swedish massage had gained a foothold in the United States. The British and French medical establishments helped legitimize Swedish massage in America as a scientific treatment for pain and disease. Doctors began to prescribe massage for illnesses and medical problems of all kinds, including fatigue and tension. People who found comfort and relief from massage began to utilize it for pleasure as well as health. Schools began to train nurses and issue certificates to prove that practitioners were skilled in the arts of the Swedish massage system.

Around 1900, however, the professional massage movement suffered a devastating blow. A report published by the British medical association noted that many schools of massage were issuing false certificates to massage students and sexual impropriety was running rampant in supposedly legitimate massage establishments. Making matters worse, claims of the curative powers of massage were being exaggerated. The American Medical Association denounced massage, paving the way for the advent of wonder drugs that became the focus of mainstream medicine. Although massage continued to be practiced by a few, the general public put their faith in scientists touting pharmacology as the cure for all human ills.

MORE THAN SKIN DEEP: THE TOUCH HEALING MOVEMENT

It wasn't until the 1960s that America began to see a revival of massage therapy, with the emergence of the holistic health movement—a movement that's still going strong today. A holistic approach to massage means treating the person as a complete organism, not just alleviating a group of symptoms. The saying that massage is more than skin deep is true. Holistic massage manipulates muscles using a variety of massage techniques to restore circulation, flexibility, and balance of energy as well as to relieve pain and discomfort. As in Chinese massage, the neuromuscular system is calmed and energy is restored. The holistic practitioner must understand anatomy and physiology and also have a feeling (either innate or learned) for life's energy.

YOU'RE PUTTY IN MY HANDS: SPA TIME

Spa means "healing waters." In Victorian times in England, around the early 1900s, healing spas were popular for ailments such as rheumatism, arthritis, and similar painful conditions. People would travel to drink from and bathe in the famed waters in spas. My hometown Harrogate in the United Kingdom is a Victorian spa town. It's no wonder I ended up in the business of healing. Spiritual and healing spas really took off in the United States in the 1960s, and since then have become a highlight of pampering, healing, and beauty. Spas are one of the fastest-growing industries today—right up there with coffeehouses!

Spas can be broken down into these basic categories, as follows:

❖ **Day spas.** These have become so popular that unless you live completely out in the sticks, you'll find one. Although day spas started out focusing on healing massage, they have gone far beyond getting rid of that nagging pain in the back. Most now focus on massage for relaxation/pleasure *and* healing. Day spas offer various facial treatments and bodywork treatments, such as deep tissue or Swedish massage.

❖ **Resort spas.** These are usually located in quality hotels and offer a large menu of services. Some of these services include the big three of (1) hydrotherapy; (2) thalassotherapy (similar to hydrotherapy, with added elements like sea salt, seaweed, and algae, which contain ingredients that help to increase blood circulation, eliminate toxins, and tone and replace minerals in the body); (3) Vichy shower (usually used after other body therapy; a massage therapist lays you on your stomach, then shoots alternating jets of pulsating water on your back). Resorts also often offer steam showers, mud wraps, salt scrubs, seaweed treatments, hot stone massage, aromatherapy massage, and/or four hands massage (which is just as it sounds, 'cause you know four hands are better than two!).

❖ **Stand-alone spas.** These are properties devoted exclusively to the spa experience. They offer full lodging, meals, spa programs, nutritional counselors, and wellness evaluations. Stand-alone spas usually offer specialized treatments, which may include mud or mineral soaks, holistic education, weight loss and management programs, nutritional counseling, and a host of delectable treats for your health, beauty, youthfulness, wellness, and recreational needs. People who attend these spas typically want a life makeover or intense healing experience and are willing to pay big bucks to get it. Massage is always a key element in their programs.

❖ **Mobile Spas.** I consider myself the leader in mobile spas, as I started Serve The Goddess over 15 years ago. Mobile spas deliver massage and spa services to the home and offices of clients, saving them the time and effort of driving to and from the spa. There's nothing better than relaxing after a massage or spa service with no traffic and no drive home. Some mobile spa owners drive around a decked-out RV, but my staff set up in clients' homes. Mobile spas are particularly popular with clients such as pregnant women and the elderly, who for health reasons can't visit a location spa.

Mobile spas cater to groups of women celebrating a special occasion, such as an upcoming wedding or birth of a baby, and offer a range of mini spa services. These women can bond with family and friends while sharing the spa experience in the same room, as there's no need for privacy. Clients can relax in familiar surroundings and create a memorable experience.

Today's spa devotee is better educated about the mind/body aspect of massage or how it affects them psychologically as well as spiritually.

The International SPA Association (ISPA) defines the spa experience as "your time to relax, reflect, revitalize, and rejoice." It's their objective to revitalize humanity ... for a price.

MASSAGE IS BEST WHEN EAST MEETS WEST

The breakthrough of travel and telecommunications opened America to the knowledge of Eastern cultures, especially Indian, Chinese, Indonesian, and Japanese societies. Some of their energizing systems include the following, based on traditional techniques from the Far East:

❖ **Thai:** a combination of yoga stretching, twisting, acupressure, and massage (done with clothes on)

❖ **Shiatsu:** the use of finger pressure on points along the meridians of the body to balance and unblock energy (done with clothes on)

❖ **Lomi Lomi:** an energetic Hawaiian massage method that uses rocking techniques

❖ **Polarity:** a technique for balancing energy through pressing and holding on different points and parts of the body

❖ **Reiki:** a form of energy exchange (passed on by a master) that aligns the body energies by placing hands gently on parts of the body in a sequence

❖ **Watsu:** a gentle underwater massage

❖ **Reflexology:** a technique involving pressing the feet or hands to bring relief to corresponding parts of the body

❖ **Indian Head Massage:** a deep scalp and neck massage especially good for relieving stress, tension, fatigue, insomnia, headaches, migraine and sinusitis

❖ **Ashiatsu:** involves a massage therapist literally walking on your back. Practitioners often hold on to specially-attached ceiling bars to maintain their balance while walking on a client's back. This type of bodywork is being heralded as a luxurious, deep-tissue massage.

With the explosion of Eastern massage ideas and practices in the United States, people began to recognize the Eastern way of understanding the body and the brain as a complete organism—rather than two separate entities—that should be treated accordingly.

Most massage therapists, including myself, do eclectic massages. I start out with some long, relaxing Swedish strokes to relax and soothe the body. But when I find a tight muscle, you'd better believe that I switch to a more intense style or even some acupressure to release the tightness, along with encouraging the recipient to do some deep breathing. What an amazing experience it can be to savor different strokes and techniques blended from all areas of the world and from all eras of time. I love that part of my work!

Now people have access to many more forms of healing massage.

Your head is probably spinning from tracing the evolution of massage over time and around the world. Remnants of ancient techniques are alive today in the many styles and approaches for healing touch. But touch is more than just a way to heal disease, overcome your aches and pains, or feel renewed. Touch is the big picture, of which couple's massage is a part.

YOUR TOUCH NOTES

❖ Massage techniques are as old as human existence.

❖ The Swedish massage system draws from ancient Chinese sources and modern physiological knowledge.

❖ Chinese and other Eastern massage techniques focus on balancing the flow of the body's energy.

❖ Massage can provide a range of healthful benefits, from improved circulation to pain management.

❖ Massage today has taken on many forms and techniques.

CHAPTER 2:
Stroking Your Way to Health

WHAT YOU'LL LEARN

❖ How massage helps your health
❖ Fighting fatigue and stress
❖ Improving circulation, immunity and oxygenation
❖ Giving your mood a boost

There aren't enough things we do in life that feel good and are good for us—but couple's massage definitely tops this list! In addition to making us feel great, couple's massage—like any kind of massage—has oodles of positive health benefits. Tiredness, negative stressors, lack of proper breathing, dead skin cells, puffy tissue, a poor immune system, and your outlook on life can all be helped with a little tender touch. Although I know you aren't necessarily stroking your honey for health, you will soon discover what good things those strokes can do for you—both physically and mentally.

A TOUCH A DAY KEEPS THE DOCTOR AWAY

The whole idea behind new age holistic cures—herbal remedies, yoga, acupuncture, meditation, and so on—is that your body has the amazing ability to heal itself. Massage, too, can be used to help your body's own healing abilities.

I am always surprised by how many people think that massages are only for the rich. Wrong! The national average price for a massage is $60.00 per hour. Still think your budget's too tight? The cost to treat yourself to a luxurious rejuvenating massage is probably less than a month's worth of those designer coffees you rely on for your wake-up call.

GETTING UNDER YOUR PARTNER'S SKIN

When you rub muscles beneath the surface of your partner's skin, your massage is improving blood flow. This gets fluids moving more efficiently, thereby cleansing the body of bacteria and waste. So in a way your massage is not only calming your partner or giving him pleasure, but also taking out his or her metabolic garbage. Aside from getting sick, not taking out the body's waste products makes people lethargic and depletes them of energy.

There is a secret communication that occurs between the person giving and the person receiving the massage. To trained fingers, for instance, tight muscles feel different than relaxed muscles do. It takes time and patience to learn this subtle language, but by explaining how massage therapy works, you'll start to get a feel for what I mean.

Do you want to send your partner a massage valentine that will bond the two of you? Ask your reclining partner to bend a leg up to the ceiling by lifting up the foot. Now let that lifted foot lean against your chest or abdomen. Put both of your hands around your partner's ankle like a human ankle bracelet. Applying pressure slowly, slide your hands up your partner's leg toward the knee. This massage movement will increase and propel blood flow toward the heart, without putting additional strain on it. You can do the same thing to your partner's arms, starting from the wrist and moving to the elbow. What a great way to heal an achy heart!

FATIGUE FIGHTER

When you're worried and stressed, chances are your body is secreting the stress hormone cortisol. This hormone prepares your body for a fight-or-flight response, which is fine if you're under attack, but not if you want to relax and get a great night's sleep.

One beautiful remedy for fatigue is right there at your fingertips—massage. When you receive a massage, pain-blocking hormones such as enkephalin and endorphins (the "feel good" hormones) are released. These counteract or block the effects of cortisol, allowing you to melt into rest and to sleep like a baby.

Now that you know that massage is a great remedy for your fatigue, don't start a fight over who's going to get the first massage or you'll get the cortisol pumping again. I know you'll figure it out, and you'll both sleep much better for having relieved your anxiety and tension. And while you're sleeping, your amazing body will regenerate itself.

> *If your partner has been suffering from insomnia, give him a massage in the evening. That way he can roll into bed and sleep the night away. Give your partner at least a half-hour massage, as it may take the body that long to de-stress. If you receive a massage in the afternoon, rest easy—a one-hour massage can be the equivalent of two or three hours of sleep.*

STRESS BUSTER

Stress causes a release of hormones that make the blood vessels narrow and constrict, which means less blood flow. This, in turn, will cause your heart to work harder and your breathing to become rapid and shallow. Digestion slows down. In fact, all body processes begin to experience dysfunction. Symptoms of stress include headaches, hypertension, depression, low back pain, and insomnia. An estimated 80 to 90 percent of illnesses are stress-induced.

Let's look at some of the common stress factors in our lives.

❖ Divorce/the end of a long-term relationship
❖ Unemployment or problems at work
❖ Pregnancy/childbirth/starting a family
❖ Moving
❖ Financial problems and serious debt
❖ Lack of love and support
❖ Family problems

We all have our unique stressors, and we handle stress in an amazing variety of ways. Couple's massage, however, seems to be a universal remedy for stress.

During a massage, your muscles relax. Your heart rate slows down, allowing a release of tension, and your breathing deepens. All of this increases the blood flow to the muscles and eliminates toxins, which have built up as a result of stress. Couple's massage is the best nonprescription drug for healing stress-related diseases.

Did you know that 70 to 90 percent of all visits to primary care physicians are for stress-related problems? Receiving regular massages prevents and treats stress.

Stress has the power to destroy relationships, but couple's massage is a great way to overcome that stress and bring couples together. One couple I know have been giving each other massages every week for six years now. They integrate massage into their lives and use it for their stress management. They hire a sitter to look after their children (two boys under the age of six). They think of their massage date as an investment in their health—it gives them time to focus on themselves and to connect with each other. Even if you become "addicted" to massaging each other, would that be such a bad thing?

Have you ever met someone who was a real pain in the neck? Stress can manifest itself in the form of a stiff neck, shoulders, and tightness in the upper chest. Tenderly massage those areas with extra care, and if there is a severe pain, see your physician.

THE RIVER OF LIFE: CIRCULATION

The circulation of blood throughout the body is essential to your health. Without that blood flow, you probably wouldn't have the capacity for being healthy at all. A good couple's massage, with its circulatory benefits, can help that blood move freely. Good circulation is the basis for all good health.

POWER BOOST: IMPROVING THE IMMUNE RESPONSE

Your lymphatic system is responsible for your body's ability to ward off infections and heal injuries. The lymphatic system doesn't have a pump of its own, like the blood system. Instead, it is dependent on the contraction and massaging of muscles to keep the lymph moving freely around the body. It's the lymph that aids in the production of white blood cells, which in turn strengthens the immune system to help fight infections. If you don't have an active lifestyle, chances are your lymphatic system is sluggish.

Studies undertaken by the Touch Research Institute in Miami found that people who received massages had higher levels of infection-fighting white blood cells. These touched bodies also showed an increased activity of so-called "natural killer cells" that attack disease.

Now you know why you have been getting those recurring colds! Never mind that flu shot. Instead you may want to give your system a boost with a couple's massage.

> *Lymphatic tissue is found in concentrated areas of the body, such as the armpit, groin, neck, knees, stomach, and in the chest. These are called lymph nodes, and they are responsible for filtering bacteria and preventing it from entering the bloodstream. If any of these areas are swollen on your partner, or if they are painful, do not massage them, as this could increase the swelling. If in doubt, check it out with your doctor.*

FILL 'ER UP: OXYGENATION

Like a squeezed sponge, a tight muscle can't hold much fluid, nor can it allow fluid to pass through it. This decreases circulation and increases the strain on your heart, robbing it of precious energy.

Massage relaxes contracted muscles and helps the circulation by pushing blood toward the heart, therefore relieving strain on this vital organ. Think of the strain of a bottleneck traffic jam—traffic simply gets stuck and can't move. Your body works the same way. An increase of circulation brings energy-producing nutrients and oxygen to your cells while carrying away metabolic waste products that make you feel listless and drained.

Ready for another bonus from your couple's massage session? Massage will increase the body's oxygen-carrying cell count, namely hemoglobin, which will help to bring more oxygen to your body's cells.

Injured muscles heal faster with massage. More and more, science is making the discovery that degenerative diseases like cancer and muscular sclerosis are anaerobic. They simply cannot survive in an oxygenated environment. You may find that through couple's massage by itself you have more energy, look more vibrant, feel better all over, and fend off infections more easily. So what are you waiting for?

> *The circulatory system is run by the heart. It transports about 10.5 pints of blood per minute when the body is resting and it pumps up to an amazing 42 pints per minute during strenuous exercise. The adult body contains about 12 pints of blood. That means that even when you are resting, all of your blood makes a complete circulation in just over a minute. Massage alone increases the blood capacity by at least 10 to 15 percent.*

SHAPING UP

In a perfect world, we would work out three times a week! But that's probably the last thing on your mind after a long day at work. And you know how sore your muscles get when you haven't worked out for a while. It is lactic acid that makes your muscles sore, and massage removes lactic acid by increasing blood circulation. Your couple's massage will also increase muscle flexibility and range of motion. Now you can get into those yoga positions you've been trying to figure out!

And if you're embarrassed about cellulite, massage (along with diet and exercise) can result in smoother skin. Massage and exercise together purify the body, increasing circulation and muscle tone.

REAL SKINNY ON SKIN

Your skin has two distinct layers: the upper layer is the epidermis, and the lower layer, under the epidermis, is the dermis. The dermis contains sweat glands, nerve endings, sensors for touch, hair follicles, and countless capillaries that supply the nutritional needs of the cells of the skin. The epidermis has no direct blood supply; it produces the hair and nails, protects and waterproofs you, and manufactures new skin cells. The skin keeps toxins out, blood in, and the body cool.

The dermal layer contains five separate sensors that detect heat, cold, pressure, pain, and light or ticklish touch. That's why a couple's massage on the skin creates so many sensations—from tickle to *ahhhhhhhhhh*.

We all know that too much sun, smog, or unhealthy food accelerates the visible signs of aging, such as dry and wrinkled skin. But did you know that massage brings more blood to the skin, resulting in a more youthful glow? With every massage stroke, you are removing toxins from the blood and delivering vital nutrients to the skin. Massage also helps reduce itchy skin by improving the function of the sebaceous gland, which lubricates and protects it from infection. Plus, a good old rubbing will accelerate the sweat glands that cool and clean the skin. As you apply oils with your couple's massage, you will be getting a dual effect, moisturizing from the outside in and the inside out.

Your skin plays an important role in your life—not just for couple's massage, but for your beauty, your health, and your whole being. Your skin requires TLC. Tender, loving care goes a long way in helping your skin thrive and glow.

Three wonderful things you can do for your skin are as follows:

❖ **Brush the skin.** *Use a skin brush on your skin before you shower or bathe. Exfoliate it on a regular basis. Daily brushing away the dead skin cells that collect on the surface will restore its healthy glow. If you'd like to know how to do dry skin brushing, click over to my blog here.* http://www.servethegoddess.com/blog/dry-skin-brushing/

❖ **Moisturize the skin.** *Use selected oils, lotions, and soaps. Avoid soaps that are detergents or that contain antimicrobial properties, as they deplete your skin of its natural protective functions. Any time you receive a couple's massage with oils, you are feeding your skin.*

❖ **Drink for the skin.** *The human body is composed of more that 60 percent water. Most Westerners consume far less water than they need. Water regulates your body temperature through sweating and exhalation from the lungs. Drink at least 8 glasses of water and your skin will show it. No more sagging, dried out, or pinched looks on those shins or upper arms!*

IT'S ALL IN YOUR HEAD: MENTAL HEALTH

How you feel emotionally and mentally has a major bearing on your physical health and well-being. Some of the leading psychologists suggest that you are what you think and feel. I agree! For example, if you have just had a fight with your oldest child about homework or found out that your business partner lied to you, you are not going to feel well. You may have tightness in your chest, a stomachache, or nonspecific pain somewhere in your body that you cannot attribute to an injury or overdoing it at the gym. But massage has the amazing ability to change your mood and your entire outlook on life. It can give your attitude a boost when you're feeling down in the dumps, and it can turn an already good day into a great one! Isn't that reason enough to keep on reading?

YOUR TOUCH NOTES

❖ Couple's massage can de-stress you.
❖ Studies show that massage contributes to better functioning of the immune system.
❖ Massage can make your skin healthier.
❖ A good massage can improve your mood.

CHAPTER 3:
Tools of the Trade

WHAT YOU'LL LEARN

❖ Choosing which oil works best
❖ Pillows for proper positioning

This chapter is going to cover the basics and then some—all the things you will need to put in your massage treasure trove to be sure that when it's time for touch, you have what I consider the necessary accessories. Of course, we all know you could just set up in the corner of your living room, lay your sweetheart down on her tummy, remove her top, and start pushing her flesh. But if you want to maximize your couple's massage experience, read on.

The line of necessities for a successful couple's massage often includes oils and something soft and comfortable to lie on. Why? Because part of the process of a couple's massage is about awakening the senses and more.

LUBING UP

The first massage essential that you'll need to get your hands on is some sort of lubricant. You're going to need something between you and your partner's body that will allow your hands to glide over the skin with smooth, relaxing movements.

Although you could certainly use lotion for massage, I have found that it's absorbed into the skin far too quickly. Instead of enjoying the process of extending pleasure, you'll be cursing under your breath as you apply more and more lotion.

Make sure that neither you nor your partner is allergic to any oils, especially peanuts or avocado, or to any of the ingredients in a massage oil mixture, such as chemicals or perfume. When in doubt, test it out. Rub a tiny bit of oil (or lotion) on your wrist and keep it on without washing for 24 hours. If irritation or a breakout occurs on the skin, don't use that particular oil.

Oil feels best if it's warmer than your body temperature. Place your bottle of oil in a pot of warm water for approximately 20 minutes to warm it up. Or splurge and buy yourself a commercial oil warmer. If your room temperature is steamy and sultry already, cut back your warm-up time to 10 minutes. Warm oil is easier to apply and feels good to both giver and receiver.

CARRIER OILS

Unlike lotion, oil will last longer, and I consider it the ideal choice for massage. Every massage movement is easier with oil that allows the hands to glide, nourishes the skin, and arouses the senses. Ready-made massage oils can be purchased at health food stores, or you can get inventive. Look around your kitchen for vegetable oils such as sunflower, peanut, or safflower oils, all of which are excellent for massage and are called "carrier oils."

Other carrier oils that you might consider include the following:

❖ **Coconut oil:** It can be purchased in economical tubs (in solid form; it liquefies at room temperature) at health food stores, and unlike most other oils or lotions, is absorbed into the skin after gentle heating. It's like food for your skin.

❖ **Apricot kernel oil:** An odorless pale yellow oil that contains minerals and vitamins and can be applied to all types of skin. This oil is very helpful to prematurely aging skin, and dry, inflamed, or sensitive skin.

❖ **Avocado oil:** Dark green in color, this carrier oil comes from the fruit itself. It contains protein, vitamins, fatty acids, lecithin, and it is odorless. Great for all skin types, especially if you have eczema or dry skin.

❖ **Grape seed oil:** (My personal choice) I recommend this oil for all types of skin. It is almost colorless and contains minerals, proteins, and vitamins. I like it because it is so light and goes a long way.

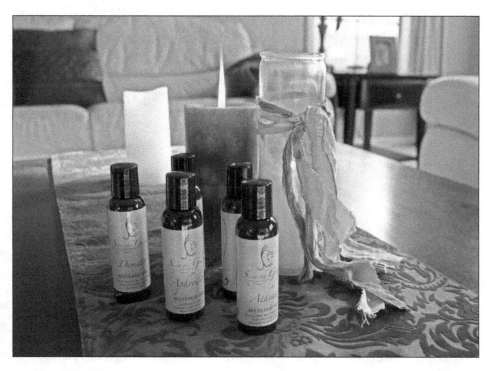

Here are some of my aromatherapy massage oils with a grape seed carrier oil. I'll discuss aromatherapy in chapter 11.
(Jaymie Garner)

❖ **Jojoba:** (This one's a little pricey.) This yellow oil comes from the jojoba bean. Because it is slightly thicker than the other oils I have described in this chapter, dilute it 10 percent with a lighter oil, such as grape seed oil. It's excellent for treating psoriasis, acne, eczema, and inflamed skin.

❖ **Sweet almond oil:** Mmm. And you thought this was a food! It is a very pale yellow color, contains minerals, vitamins, and is rich in proteins. It comes from the kernel of the almond and helps relieve itching, soreness, inflammation, and dryness.

❖ **Wheat germ oil:** It is a yellow-orange color and needs to be diluted 10 percent with a lighter oil, such as sweet almond or grape seed oil. It contains vitamins, minerals, and proteins, and is used especially for prematurely aging skin, psoriasis, and eczema, although it is suitable for all skin types.

❖ **Vitamin E:** Although it's very thick and extremely expensive, vitamin E is great to use on your or your partner's face, which is more delicate than the rest of the skin and requires only a thin coating of oil.

Putting oil of any kind on the face can result in acne or other eruptions or irritations on the skin. I recommend using apricot kernel oil or sweet almond oil on the face, as they are evenly balanced, which is important, as the skin on the face is usually a combination of dry, oily, and normal skin types.

Once you've found a carrier oil that you like working with, you can add an essential oil to it, the fragrance of which will spice up your couple's massage. Mixing essential oils with carrier oils can create different effects on your partner, from relaxing to invigorating, depending on the combination. I discuss essential oils in detail in chapter 11.

The quantity of oil you use is important. If you add too much oil, your hands will skid all over your partner's body and you will be unable to make proper contact—too little oil and you will end up making uneven, jerky movements.

To aid in getting just the right amount of oil, pour your massage oil into a plastic squeeze bottle. When you're ready to begin the massage, pour just enough oil to cover the hollow of your palm. You can always add more if you feel the skin drying out. It is always easier to add more than to mop up too much. Don't add oil to the whole body at once—you can add oil to other parts of the body as you progress.

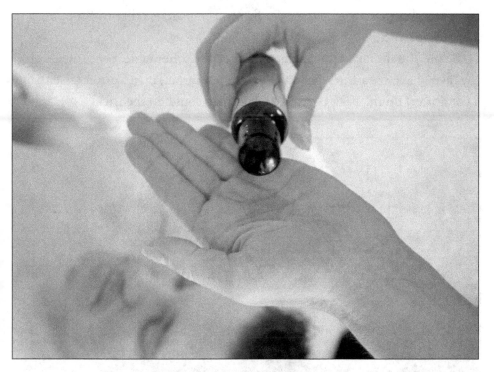

Pour a quarter-size amount of oil into the palm of your hand first. You can always add more as you need it. (Jaymie Garner)

You can use any of the above-mentioned carrier oils for the feet. However, go lightly with oils on the soles of the feet, so that the person receiving the massage doesn't slip when he gets up to walk and to minimize carpet stains.

If you are worried about staining sheets or clothes with massage oil, you can purchase nonstaining massage lotions and oils that the professionals use. These are available at massage supply stores.

MORE CUSHION FOR THE PUSHIN'

The first place most people think to give a massage is on their bed. However, most mattresses are too soft and pliable, not offering any support for the giver. For a couple's massage you'll need a firm, strong surface that will support you and your partner.

Before you decide on the kitchen table or the coffee table, assess their stability. If you have extra-thick padding under your carpet, then a duvet (essentially, a comforter) on the floor covered with a sheet could do the trick.

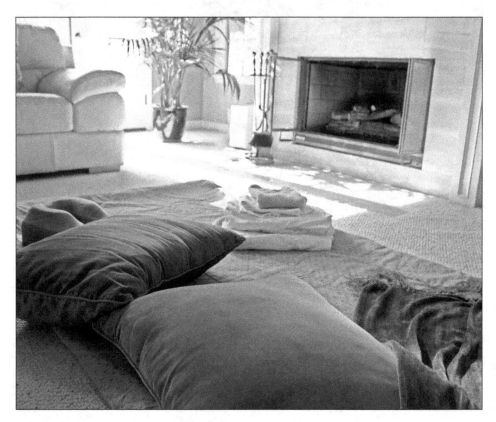

Place a pillow behind your knees for comfort.

(Jaymie Garner)

A double-size futon mattress will also work, but of course there has to be enough room for the person giving the massage to move around.

If you have a U-Shaped Neck Pillow that you use for travel, it will make an ideal face cradle to support your partner's head and neck during your couple's massage. For extra comfort, invest in the memory foam one. To prevent oil stains, cover the neck pillow with a pillow case. Place the neck pillow at the head of the mattress or mattress pad and ask them to place their face on it. Your partner will soon discover this pillow is more comfortable than lying with their head turned to one side.

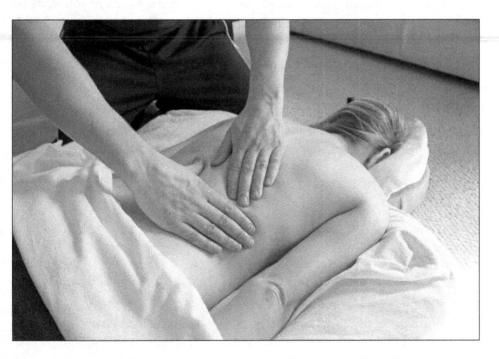

Place a U-Shaped Neck Pillow at the head of the mattress for your partner's comfort.
(Jaymie Garner)

The most comfortable massage surface for both giver and receiver is one that is firm but has a pliant surface. It supports the back nicely and doesn't rock or sway when pressure is applied on the body. The best type of surface allows room to move around the massage area, plus has a well-padded surface for knees.

Be wise about what you use for your massage platform. Avoid accidental injuries by using a stable flooring, tables, or a couch, and don't take chances with anything that may wobble and break. The sheer weight of your body and the added pressure of the massage itself can be too much strain for many tables. As with anything that you choose for pleasure, always put safety first!

If you use a table, make sure it isn't too low, so that the partner giving the massage doesn't have to hunch over. If the table is too high, you won't be able to apply enough pressure with your body, and believe me when I tell you that you are going to tire easily when only using pressure from your hands. Being at just the right height will propel you into lasting action.

Determining the appropriate height for your massage surface is simple. Stand next to the table with your arms down by your side and make a fist. If your fist is level with the surface, then it's just right. If it's not, then you need to adjust the height.

GOING PRO

If you find that you really like giving and receiving couple's massages, you may want to go all out and invest in a professional massage table. Expect to pay around $250 for a basic table with adjustable legs and a face cradle, which is a donut-shaped extension of the table where the receiver's head rests. I recommend the fine tables from Living Earth Crafts, EarthLite, and Oakworks. They all come with a manufacturer's guarantee, and you can buy them in massage supply stores. You can even buy a carrying case if you plan on taking your table on that Hawaiian vacation.

Not only does a massage table enable you to massage while standing up (which is less tiring than kneeling), but your partner will also be more comfortable with her head cradled in that funny donut hole. Single (twin) sheets fit most massage tables. When you're not using the table, you can fold it up and stash it under the bed or in the closet. Pretty neat, eh?

SHORT ON TIME

If you're short on time, you can do just a foot massage or a scalp massage. You can ask your sweetheart to join you on the sofa and you won't need all the props. I'll cover the massage routine for the feet in chapter 7.

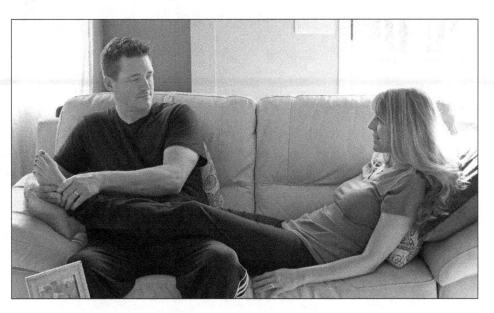

If you're short on time, a 15- to 20-minute foot massage does the trick
(Jaymie Garner)

YOUR TOUCH NOTES

❖   Oil is the best lubricant for your massage.
❖   Your massage platform should give you support and your partner comfort.
❖   Pillows protect your knees so you won't tire easily.
❖   A professional massage table is worth the investment.

CHAPTER 4:
The ABCs of Massage

WHAT YOU'LL LEARN

❖   Keeping your approach warm and gentle
❖   Making sure your body is ready for a massage
❖   The dos and don'ts of massage
❖   The art of taking your time

It's time to clear the air about how difficult it is to give good couple's massage…
It's easy!

Even if you said to us, "I'm all thumbs," you could still give your partner an incredible experience—the thumbs are great massage tools! All you need is the desire to give your partner pleasure and plenty of good old-fashioned patience. I'll take care of the rest.

In this chapter, I demonstrate a few essential tips and techniques so that you and your partner can begin to explore the path to pleasure. Just remember this: Always be caressing and gentle, and let your hands do the talking. I'll explore the material covered in this chapter in much more detail later in the book, but here you'll find enough information to get you started.

"A" IS FOR APPROACH

Your approach will create the mood you want for the couple's massage. Imagine two scenarios: In the first, you say sharply, "Hey! Do you want a massage? I've got 20 minutes, so hurry up." In the second, you gently ask, "Would you like me to make you feel relaxed and warm all over? Climb into bed and close your eyes…" In the first situation, you've probably already made your partner tense, and that's the last thing you want to do when initiating a couple's massage. Instead your approach, or invitation, should already begin the process of relaxing your partner, as the second scenario demonstrates.

How you approach your couple's massage partner depends upon your moods, his or her availability, and the setting. It's even possible that your partner may need some coaxing or cajoling to focus on what he or she wants from a massage. Is he tired from swinging a golf club all afternoon? Is she anxious from studying for the bar exam all day? Is he moody from just getting the axe at work, or is she pouting because she's having a bad hair day again?

> *Think of your partner as a cat: No cat owner in her right mind would grab her kitty, brush it with a wire brush, then expect it to stay on her lap purring with pleasure. Any cat worth his sardines would lash out with his razor-sharp claws, then run off and hide. Approach your partner in the same way you would approach a kitty: gently and sweetly.*

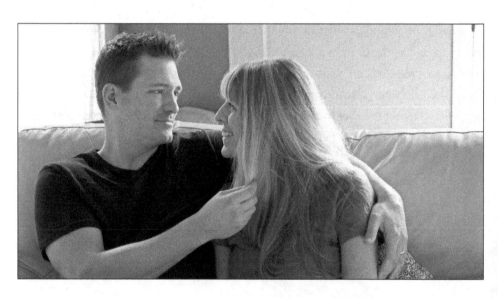

Approach your partner sweetly and invite her to a couple's massage session.
(Jaymie Garner)

Once you've gently invited your partner to enjoy the touch of your hands, you need to make sure those hands are ready to touch your partner. Warm your hands—you can do this by rubbing them together or running them under hot tap water and then drying them. Likewise, any oils that you use should be warmed before you apply them. (I'll be discussing room ambiance in chapter 9; I discussed massage surfaces and carrier oils in chapter 3.)

TAKE IT ALL OFF?

You will want to decide what level of undress feels comfortable for you both. How much or little you bare really depends on what you both prefer. There's nothing wrong with wearing sweats or hiding behind/under huge towels or wearing workout gear.

"B" IS FOR BODY ETIQUETTE

When it comes to body etiquette, think clean. Here are some basic places on your body to inspect and upgrade if necessary:

❖ **Clean up your act.** Step one is getting clean. That may mean a quick shower or a long pre-massage bath. Your choice!

❖ **Nails.** Make sure that you trim your nails. File them so that they are smooth, and then test them on your inner wrist to check for jagged edges or hangnails. If you have long nails and don't want to cut them, practice stroking your partner in a way that won't hurt him. The simpler and shorter the better.

❖ **Whiskers.** Guys, listen up: You don't want to leave your couple's massage partner with razor burn instead of heart palpitations of love, do you? If you have a beard or mustache, make sure it's trimmed; otherwise, shave away that five o'clock shadow or two days' worth of stubble. Of course, I will excuse your stubble if you are growing a beard and your partner is aware!

❖ **Basic Oral Hygiene.** Imagine that you're preparing to give your partner the touch treatment of a lifetime. Just as you approach his head to stroke his cheeks and temples, he opens his mouth and breathes day-old pizza and beer breath into your face. Ugh! The moral of our little story is this: Brush your teeth, use a mouthwash or a tongue scraper if needed, and floss daily. If you haven't noticed that dentistry has moved out of medieval times, you need to book that appointment for a cleaning, too.

❖ **Hands.** Rough hands require TLC before you put finger to flesh. If you are a car mechanic or a rodeo master, you may have to work to get smooth skin. Most people will just have to make some minor adjustments to have hands that feel good to the touch. Use hand creams on a regular basis, and if you really want to do this well, do a good hand soaking. Soaking in a solution of sea salts will let your skin shed those old crusty particles that make it rough or dry.

❖ **Elbows.** Use the same sea salt solution that you used with your hands to soften those crusty elbows. Or try a loofah mitt to scrub the nobs into submission.

Try this recipe for smooth hands:

The day before giving your couple's massage, soak your hands for 20 minutes in saltwater, using sea salts and warm water as your solution. You can add essential oils, such as lavender or tea tree, to the solution if you want to. Lavender is relaxing and the tea tree is a natural antibiotic—good for healing cuts and little tears on the skin surface. Rub your hands together with the sea salt, which causes friction and helps to remove dead skin on both the inside and outside skin, letting the oils absorb. (You can also do this to your feet.) Apply a hand moisturizer to replenish the natural oils that you have sloughed away.

After applying the moisturizer, wear a pair of cotton gloves to keep the gooey, wet stuff you've applied on your hands rather than on furniture, your clothes, or whatever else you touch.

If you like going to a salon for your beauty and skin treatments, ask for the paraffin hand dip, which feels weird at first (like, is this how aliens feel?) but then if you can surrender to it, it feels great. You'll look mahvelous, darling, too! You can also now buy home paraffin kits.

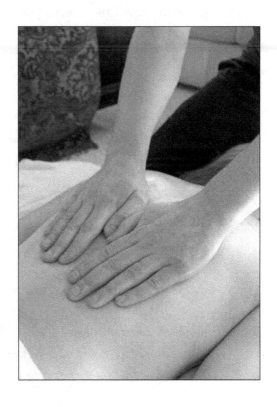

Trim your nails short; no one wants to feel your nails digging in during your massage. (Jaymie Garner)

"C" IS FOR COMMITMENT

You've got the relaxing music turned down low, the massage oil is warm in your hands, and you're ready to make your partner's head spin with pleasure.

Now don't spoil the mood by thinking about the time. Set aside a few hours so that you can make the most of the experience. Although you shouldn't expect anything after your couple's massage other than the good vibes of having given or received pleasure, let me be candid: A great couple's massage can help you bond on a deeper level.

Choose whatever amount of time feels right. You'll be shocked at how quickly time passes when you are giving couple's massage—especially for the person on the receiving end!

Here are some more tips to make your time together even better:

❖ As you are caressing your partner's body, imagine that you are actually massaging yourself. Would you want patient attentiveness given to your body?

❖ Listen to the sounds your partner makes, and distinguish between the *oohs*, *ahs*, and *ouches*. If you remain quiet, you will learn more about your partner by giving couple's massage than you could learn by exchanging a thousand words. The touch of love says so much more than words could ever say, and if your partner starts purring, you know it's right.

❖ Always caress with long, slow, gentle strokes, and enjoy.

Set a quiet timer or use one of our CDs to let you know when time's up. Or invest in one of those gorgeous and soothing Zen clocks that let you record your own voice, or that smartphone timer ring with a pleasant Tibetan chime.

COUPLE'S MASSAGE DOS AND DON'TS

Here are some other things to keep in mind to make the most of your couple's massage:

Do…

❖ Ask your partner if he has any sore muscles before you begin.

❖ Find out if your partner has any ticklish areas, such as feet or midsection. If so, avoid a light touch in those areas.

❖ Be sensitive to your partner's response to the massage. If she starts drifting off to la-la land, let her go there.

❖ Relax before you dive into touch. Breathe a little, listen to some soothing tunes, or even sip some calming tea, such as valerian root or a chamomile.

❖ Be responsive to your partner's needs. If he isn't in the mood to give you a massage, be the giver this time. Same thing for if she's not ready to reciprocate—relax and give it a rest.

❖ Let your strokes flow into one another with no abrupt endings. Keeping both hands on the body at all times is your anchor for staying connected to your lucky massage recipient.

❖ Give equal time to each of the 10 body zones (see chapters 6 and 7 for more on these). The legs, arms, and shoulders should all get the same amount of your amazing touch.

Don't…

❖ Talk too much. If you have to talk, speak softly.

❖ Jump right into a massage. You wouldn't jump into a pool of water without first testing the temperature, would you? Ask your partner if he or she is too cold or hot. Men are usually warmer than women are, but there are exceptions to the rule.

❖ Comment on how tight muscles might feel. If you come across a tight muscle, let your hands do the talking. Work around the tight area, giving it a little more love and attention.

❖ Pour oil directly onto the body. This can be a bit of a shock, and it isn't as comforting as your hands gently gliding onto your partner's body with warm oil.

❖ Eat a heavy meal before receiving a massage. This can cause mild to severe discomfort while lying on your stomach. Instead eat a light meal a few hours before the massage.

My massage clients sometimes complain that other massage therapists tell them, during a massage, that their muscles are tight or say something such as "Oh my God! How can you walk around with such tight shoulders?" This sort of comment will only succeed in creating tension between you and your partner. If you want your couple's massage to be a pleasurable experience, focus on the positive. Negative talk only interferes with relaxation.

SLOW DOWN, YOU MOVE TOO FAST!

It takes mental training, the right attitude, and a commitment to share a couple's massage. The key? Slowing it all down. If you were to take just one piece of advice from this book, it should be this: Take your time. Stop the frenzy. Stop the multitasking.

Try the following suggestions for slowing down:

❖ **Breathe.** To avoid pain, to endure the pressures of a certain massage technique or placement on the body, to clear the tensions of the day, or to be in a mindful state, breathing is a key element. Breathing helps you to focus on pleasurable sensations, keeps the attention on the body, and promotes good circulation.

❖ **Use music as audio wallpaper.** Use music to set the mood, keep the pace, enhance the romance, and soothe jangled nerves. You can select music for pepping up the energy or easing into a slower pace for this special time together.

❖ **Light and darkness.** Too much light in a massage area can be distracting. In chapter 9, I discuss selecting and preparing the right locations and settings for your couple's massage. Having the proper lighting will help you get in the mood for massage.

❖ **Time management.** Oh boy. I know how challenging it can be to take the time out for play. Managing time is one of the greatest challenges of today's insanely busy world. Whew. No wonder your back is aching for a massage of any kind.

Move more slowly, be mindful, and I guarantee your life is going to improve. So is your personal life.

Let yourself indulge in time for couple's massage and make it count. You'll reap more than just rewards, I promise.

YOUR TOUCH NOTES

❖ Your approach to couple's massage will determine its outcome.
❖ Get squeaky clean before you lie down on the massage table.
❖ Set aside enough time so that you can both enjoy the experience.
❖ Slowing down is a key to successful couple's massage.

CHAPTER 5:
Different Strokes for Different Folks

WHAT YOU'LL LEARN

❖ The incredible human hand's design for touch
❖ Using other body parts as massage tools
❖ How to reduce strain and avoid pain
❖ Mastering the four basic strokes
❖ Determining your intensity, style, and type of touch

Did you ever think that the craggy, nubby thing called your elbow would turn into a cute massage tool? Knees, elbows, chins, forearms—even foreheads—no part of your body is going to seem the same after you read this chapter!

There's more to massage than most people think. In addition to mastering the stroke itself, you need to know how much pressure to apply and what kind of rhythm to use. And if you don't position your and your partner's bodies properly during the massage, neither one of you will be relaxed or comfortable.

Are you ready for the inside scoop on what it *really* takes to give a good massage?

NEED A HAND?

Open your hands and take a close look at them. If the inside of your hands is facing you, the heel of your hand is the bottom fleshy part that meets the wrist and thumb. The area below the fingers is known as the mound of the hand, and it's just like the ball of your tootsie. Both the heel and the mound are essential massage tools. The side of your hand can also be instrumental for certain massage strokes, as can the flat surface in the center of your hand under your mound, which is known as the palm.

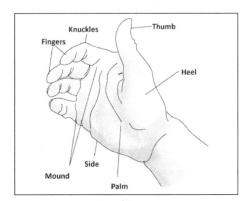

If I didn't know better, I'd say that the human hand was designed for giving couple's massage! (Vladimir Cebu)

If I didn't know better, I'd say that hands were created specifically for giving couple's massages. Even if you just rely on your knuckles—both the ones at the bottom of the fingers and in the fingers themselves—you can propel your lucky massage partner into bliss. Knuckling is a good way to relieve pressure and create oh-so-pleasant sensations.

Equally essential to massage are the fingers—they're handy helpers that are perfect when you want to target smaller areas or do more delicate work. You can use all of your fingers together like a gripping device for squeezing and kneading, or you can use the fingertips for a stroke that's similar to finger painting. Your fingers can really push deeply into the flesh to release tension, relax the muscles, or even just prod and tickle.

And don't forget your fabulous thumb—it's a little tool all its own for getting those tricky areas between the shoulder blades, the neck, and supplementing the work that your fingers do.

DON'T FORGET ABOUT YOUR FEET AND ELBOWS

Although hands really are the perfect massage tools, other body parts can be used to create wonderful sensations and to give your hands a break when they get tired. For instance, anything you can do with your hands and fingers, you can also do with those feet of yours, just like the Shiatsu and Thai massage masters. Your heels can push and prod your partner's derriere, or you can sit behind him and push your tootsies into his aching, tired shoulders. *Ahhhh.* You as the giver will feel the delight of stretching out your gams while your fortunate partner will be ooohing and ahhing as he lets go of all that tension carried in the tops of his shoulders.

If your legs are strong, you can use your knees to create powerful sensations quite effortlessly. Making sure you're not putting your full weight on his body, press your knees into your partner's buttocks. Move those knees gently up the sides of his rear end. (If you get really good at this, you may be an applicant for a new job at the Shiatsu center near you.) It's a nice way to say "I love you" without words.

> *Never, never put pressure on a bone, especially the spinal column. And even if your weights are evenly matched, be cautious about using the full weight of your body on your partner. In particular, avoid putting a lot of pressure or weight on the areas above the waist on the back and front of the body, where the organs such as the kidneys are situated.*

The most common complaint I get from women about their partner's massage is that he gives up after five minutes and loses interest. For men it's that their partner is not strong enough. I hear all the time, *Don't your hands get tired?* Read on to see why your stamina does not come from your hands alone.

LESS STRAIN, MORE GAIN

Positioning, or how and where you place your body while giving a massage, is probably one of the most important things I can show you how to do. The more you can do to minimize your strain, the more pleasure you and your partner will feel. Believe it or not, if you just use your hands or fingers, you're going to run out of steam pretty quickly, left to wonder what the heck you did wrong or to despise the act of couple's massage. That's the last thing I want to happen. Instead I want you to feel great and make it last a long time.

There are a variety of positions you can get into while giving a massage. You may find it easier, depending on each situation, to stand, sit, kneel, straddle, or lie next to your partner. Each position has its limitations. If you are straddling your partner's body, for example, you can reach only certain areas of the body. If you are kneeling near his lower back, you'll probably have to scoot down to reach his lower legs and move up to reach his shoulders, and you'll only be able to reach one side of his flanks, ribs, or legs.

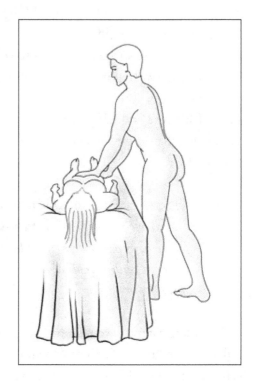

When standing, keep your back straight, and whenever necessary bend your knees rather than your back. Keep your feet apart for a firm base. (Vladimir Cebu)

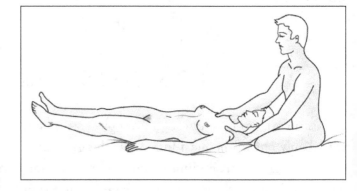

When sitting, keep your back straight, and don't hunch over. (Vladimir Cebu)

When straddling your partner, keep your back straight, and avoid scrunching or curving your spine. You'll probably want to alternate this position with other positions. Don't collapse on your partner while straddling across him or her. (Vladimir Cebu)

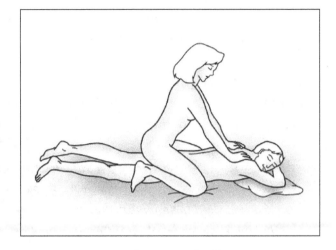

Use a pillow under your knees and behind your calves for support and comfort when kneeling. Keep your spine straight, body upright, and move your whole body with your massage strokes. (Vladimir Cebu)

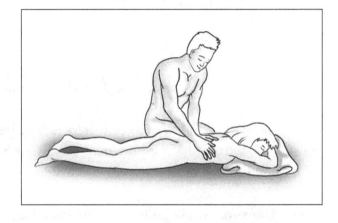

You are limited in where you can reach when lying down. This is perhaps the most intimate position of all, letting your body touch his, like spoons, or facing your partner's body. (Vladimir Cebu)

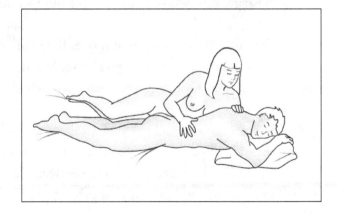

You will have to move yourself around to access the full body of your partner. Standing beside or at the ends of your partner, especially if you use a professional massage table, will help you to reach with longer strokes. Experiment with the different alignments, and you will eventually discover your favorite way to give touch. You may even decide to use them all, integrating the many ways to share touch and intimacy on different occasions.

> *The best way to avoid tiring yourself out or putting too much strain on your hands, fingers, legs, or any other part of your body is to vary what you do. You may want to push the flesh with your fingertips for a while, then switch to knuckling, or kneel into it or use your forearm. Think about all of the possible ways that you can stimulate a response in your partner, and figure in all of your own body parts that you can use.*

ALL THE RIGHT ANGLES

It's important to follow these principles for angling yourself as the giver of the couple's massage. It's not just about using your hands. Hands and fingers are the extensions of other movements and abilities.

- ❖ **Use your whole body, not just your hands.** When you conduct a massage, your whole body moves from its center.

- ❖ **Use your hips to help you move.** If you are reaching across the body, let your hips sway to take you there, Maintain a straight spine as much as you can, elongating your back as much as possible.

- ❖ **Support those knees.** Using a rolled-up towel or small pillow on the backside of your knees when you are in kneeling mode will keep your feet from falling asleep. Staying comfortable will allow you to focus on your partner and not on your aches and pains.

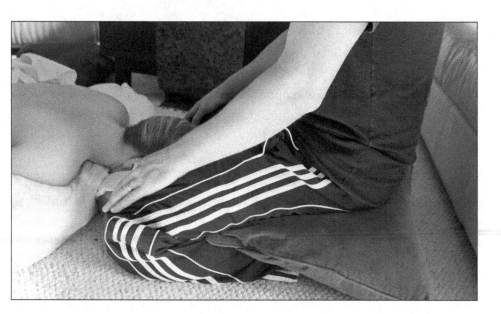

This pillow will support your knees.

(Jaymie Garner)

This diagram demonstrates proper wrist placement for various strokes and positions.

(Vladimir Cebu)

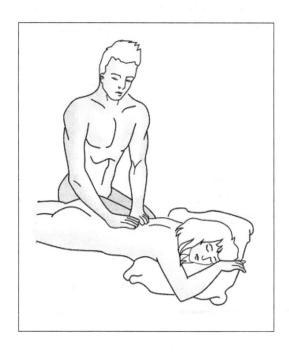

❖ **Make sure that your wrists are placed just above and in the same angle as your hand for proper touch.** Lean into the angle of your hand with your body weight placed above the hands. If you follow the motions and movements of your hands with your whole body, you will avoid strain and stay in good alignment. Bottom line: Don't rest all of your weight on your hands, but do lean into your hands to let your weight flow with their every move.

❖ **Make sure that your shoulders are relaxed.** Good shoulder posture is a must, otherwise you're the one who's going to need the massage!

❖ **Keep your hands loose and relaxed.** Use all the many parts of your hands, switching from the teeny little pads at the tips of your fingers to the palms, mounds, sides, and thumbs. Or use a tennis ball to release built-up tension and muscle tiredness. Hands do tire, so give them a rest now and then.

There are times when a light touch is called for, such as to show the more playful parts of your personality. Other situations command a deeper probe, whether it's to create relaxation, help in the release of built-up tension in the muscles, or to change the mood of the massage. And, by the way, changing intensity from one stroke to another may also help you focus better.

If your hands ever get tired while you're giving a massage, then you're not using proper body alignment. Relying on your hands alone is a surefire route to disaster. Rely more on your body weight to create pressure, rather than pushing with your fingers or thumbs.

Let's face it, if you're a 90-pound woman trying to give a pleasant massage to a 300-pound partner, you're not going to get far with your hands alone. And if heavy Harry is to massage you, he'd better position himself carefully to find the proper leverage to avoid crushing your bones.

STROKE IT!

Now that you know how to position yourself to get the most out of your body, it's time to learn some basic strokes. I recommend four basic strokes that you can easily learn without going to massage school. I'll refer to these same four strokes—and variations on them—throughout the rest of this book.

In addition to describing the strokes, I'll also suggest what kind of *rhythm* to strive for when using them. However, you shouldn't be afraid to try your own rhythms as well.

Rhythm *means how fast or slowly you rub, stroke, push, or knead.*

ROLL IT

Let's start with the first stroke—I call it "roll it." This is a long, gliding stroke that soothes the muscles and relaxes the body while also increasing circulation. You can use it on most parts of the body, but it is particularly effective on the back, chest, arms, and legs.

To perform this stroke, push using the whole hand—from the heels of your hands through to your fingers—and on the return, pull back through the fingers to the heel of the hands. Repeat. You can perform this stroke up and down the length of the body or across it.

Try to keep your rhythm slow and languid when rolling it—these strokes feel better the slower you go. You don't want to rush. Don't just do one or two strokes and then stop; instead, repeat the stroke 15 or so times to get your partner purring. Conjure up a slow waltz in your mind to set the rhythm of this one—slow, easy, and gliding.

51

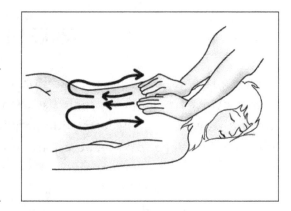

"Roll-it's" long, smooth strokes are sure to make your partner sigh as she/he starts to unwind.
(Vladimir Cebu)

A variation of roll it uses the same movement, but instead of a long stroke, it's horizontal—like finger painting, but I promise that it's more fun when you're "finger painting" the back of your partner. This stroke is great for nagging aches in neck and back muscles. For variety, try speeding your stroke up a bit, making it peppy.

Use your fingers to make small, circular, rubbing motions along the sides of the spine and between the shoulder blades. If you don't get a sigh here from your partner, I'd be surprised.

KNEAD IT

The second stroke is "knead it," and it's a classic Swedish massage maneuver (see chapter 1 for more on Swedish massage). This stroke feels great on the shoulders, thighs, and buttocks, where you can easily lift and gently squeeze the muscles.

To perform the knead-it stroke, lift and squeeze the muscle between your thumbs and fingers using a single hand or alternating between both hands. You can use your knuckles to push into the flesh where the muscle is tighter.

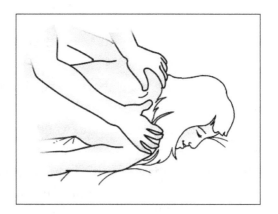

"Knead it" involves lifting and squeezing the muscles between your fingers and thumb. (Vladimir Cebu)

Move your hands in a figure-8 pattern while kneading the flesh. Try to keep a moderate tempo—faster than the languid movements of roll it, but not so fast that your movements are jerky.

I discuss oils and lotions you can use for your couple's massage in chapter 3, but if you don't have any on hand, grab some massage oil from your local health food store. Steady, though—use just enough oil to fit in the cup of your hand. It's easier to add more if you feel the skin drinking up the oil than to mop it up if you use too much.

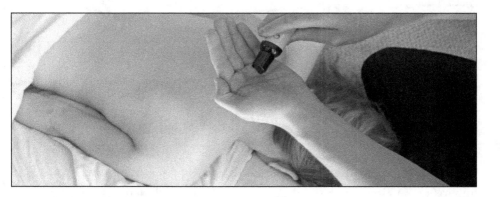

Pour just enough oil to fit into your hand. (Jaymie Garner)

53

TAP IT

"Tap it" is just like it sounds—tapping and beating on the skin using light to medium pressure. The stroke, which is also known as tapotement in the Swedish massage system, works wonders on the back, shoulders, and feet. Use your fingers for a lighter tap and your soft fist for a firmer tap or beat. It can also be used on the chest, legs, and buttocks.

Start lightly and increase pressure with feedback from your partner. Use the fingers for a lighter tap and a soft fist for a firmer tap or beat. Beat like a drum—you choose the tempo.

You can vary the pressure of the "tap it" stroke and even use your fists or knuckles instead of your fingers.
(Vladimir Cebu)

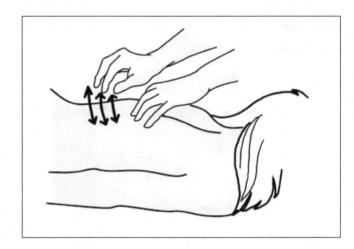

BRUSH IT

"Brush it" is a whisper of a stroke, like using a feather. Slowly trail your fingers, using alternate hands, up your partner's back, legs, chest, and arms. You can use the brush-it stroke up and down the length of the body or across it.

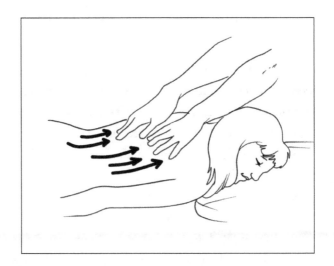

"Brush it" involves long, slow strokes up and down or across the body, using your fingers, hands, or any other body part. (Vladimir Cebu)

Be generous with your touch when massaging your partner and listen to her responses. If she is sighing with pleasure, that's probably a sign that she wants you to continue with that stroke. Always remember to stay with slow, rhythmic strokes—not fast and jerky ones that can interrupt the flow. Be creative and gentle.

PLAY AROUND

For now, play around with these strokes until you're comfortable with them. In chapters 6 and 7 I'll run through some complete massages step by step—including how to position yourself to get the most out of your movements.

Even though I have walked you through some basic strokes and suggested where to use them, you should feel free to develop your own style as you go. If you only want to do a part of the body in one sitting, fine. If you want to go faster or use your own strokes on body parts, you may discover a whole new way of touch on your own. As long as you don't push too hard on sore places, put pressure on the bony regions, or crash on your partner with a 10-ton force, you can play with this all you want.

YOUR PERSONAL PLEASURE AND PRESSURE POINTS

Now that you know *how* to touch your partner, let's take a minute or two to consider *where* to touch her. In other words, you'll want to figure out where on your partner's body touch feels pleasurable, where it's ticklish, where it hurts, and where it's a turn-on.

Different areas of the body feel touch differently. Here are some standard sensations that people have when touched on various parts of their bodies:

❖ **Tickle points.** Tickling is fine, when that's what you want—a gentle tickle can relax or arouse. But the deep poking kind of tickling should typically be avoided during a massage. Common tickle points are the bottom of the feet, under the arms (underarm), and the ribs.

❖ **Relaxation points.** These are the areas on the body that when touched induce a sigh of relief from the receiver, even a sound of *ahhhh*. They make you feel good. They let you let go. They open up your ability to release tension, which is probably why everyone wants to be touched on those points. Think about how good it feels to have your shoulders or elbows touched, for instance. In addition to the shoulders and elbow, common relaxation points are the back of the neck, scalp, back, hands, and feet.

❖ **Pressure points.** In most Eastern medicine systems, there are designated points and pathways (often called meridians) that carry energy to and from the organs. If you've ever had acupuncture, reflexology, or an acupressure massage, you've had your points pushed. Many people believe that massaging these points can heal the body.

SHOW AND TELL

Because you want to achieve the desired mood during your massage, it's important that you and your partner are aware of what parts of your bodies evoke different sensations. Talk to your partner about where those three types of points—tickle, relaxation, and pressure—are on your bodies.

> *Do you want to see tension melt away from your partner's shoulders? Here's a technique you can use. Have him lie face down, and then rest your hands on his shoulders. Sink your thumbs into the shoulders directly under the earlobes. If his muscles are tight, this might hurt, so ease into it and tell your partner to breathe deeply as you push. Move your hands to the side about an inch and repeat, continuing the entire process about four times. This technique releases tension in that famous tension-holding muscle called the trapezius. From there you can move down the side of the spine, hitting points about an inch on either side of the spine.*

HANDLE WITH CARE

If you touch a point on your partner's body where she says it hurts, proceed carefully. Although some pain does feel good, it's also a signal that something's not right. So if you do hit a pain point and your partner tells you it's too much, ease up. If she's enjoying a little ouch, then go for it. It's important to find your own balance, as the last thing you want is to cause pain or harm during a massage.

You'll also want to avoid applying too much, if any, pressure on other parts of the body. No-no's may include the following:

Spine

Ribs

Anklebones

Eyes

Kidneys (just above the waistline on the back)

Stomach and abdomen

Carotid artery (just to the side of the neck)

Breastbone (that part between the breasts in both men and women)

Diaphragm

Clavicle (collarbone)

Wrists

Elbows

I've mentioned this before, and it's worth repeating: Avoid leaning on your partner to support your own weight. Imagine your sweetie placing 220 pounds of body weight on that delicate floating rib—talk about ouch! If you are on the receiving end and your partner is applying too much pressure or is using you as an armchair, tell him to stop. Couple's massage is meant to be for pleasure.

FIND YOUR FLAIR

When it comes to couple's massage styles, you are going to evolve your own. Styles for touching can be as different as hairstyles. The best way to discover how well your hands work on your partner's body is to practice. Don't be afraid to try out all of the methods, approaches, and techniques I mention in this book until you find the one or more that suit you.

Once you find your primary touch style, indulge yourself in it. Really jump in. Don't judge what you do or how you are doing it. As long as you stay focused on what your hands are doing and your connection with your partner, you'll be fine.

You may discover, for instance, that you feel more confident or even do a better job when pushing deeply into the tissues, making you more of a deep tissue massage-giver. Or you may like the long slow strokes of the Swedish method. You may even develop a combination of strokes, rhythms, and intensities or special movements on your partner that can change with time or that will become a style that is uniquely yours. For example, you may like to make little butterfly wings with your fingers on her flesh or pull on your lover's earlobes, or even use your mouth more that your fingers. Go for it!

YOUR TOUCH NOTES

❖ The hand makes a wonderful massage tool, as do your other body parts.
❖ Proper positioning and alignment reduce body strain.
❖ The four basic strokes are roll it, knead it, tap it, and brush it.
❖ Avoid all forms of harmful and painful touch.
❖ You can develop your own unique style for touch.

CHAPTER 6:
Facedown, Back Up: Massage Round #1

WHAT YOU'LL LEARN

❖ Final pre-massage checklist
❖ The five zones of the body facedown
❖ Massaging the five zones

In this chapter and the next one, I suggest a sample massage routine. Even though I provide steps for you to follow, you should know by now that I strongly encourage you to go with the flow and do whatever seems right at the moment. Don't be afraid to try different strokes—even using parts of the body besides your hands. This step-by-step massage should be your starting point—to give you an idea of the basics—so have fun with it!

I begin the massage routine with the receiver's body lying face down. In chapter 7, I flip the body over and stroke the face-up side.

Note: Although I use the female pronoun throughout this chapter for ease of reference, either gender can be the first to receive the massage. For the sake of fairness, I'll shift to the male pronoun in chapter 7.

YOUR PRE-MASSAGE CHECKLIST

Like a pilot preparing for takeoff, you'll want to make sure that you and your "passenger" are prepared for your journey. Here's a pre-massage checklist for you to run through.

❖ **Comfort:** Begin by making sure your partner is comfortable. Does she have enough pillows for support, such as under her feet, or a face cradle to keep her head supported?

❖ **Temperature:** Is she warm enough? Make sure the temperature is set to her comfort level. If you get too hot or cold, you know that you can easily strip down or add layers of clothing to warm yourself up.

❖ **Alignment:** Make sure that she is lying facedown in a straight line.

❖ **Trouble spots:** Ask your partner if she has any injuries or sore places on her body. Avoid touching the injured areas and spend more time massaging the sore parts.

❖ **Grounding:** Prepare yourself both physically and emotionally. In chapter 12, I'll discuss setting your intention, including how your thoughts and feelings can get transmitted through your hands. Now is the time to sit quietly and to take some deep breaths while you set your intentions for your couple's massage experience.

❖ **Warm hands:** Before you touch a molecule of her skin, rub your hands together to warm them up. No one wants icy fingers and hands on their flesh.

❖ **Lube up:** Have your oil ready to apply. Put a dab of oil about the size of a quarter on your own palm. Rub your hands together. Remember, never pour oil directly onto your partner's skin.

❖ **Protect your knees:** Remember to get a soft pillow to put between your feet and your bottom if you plan to kneel during the massage (which is my recommended position throughout this sample massage). It really helps!

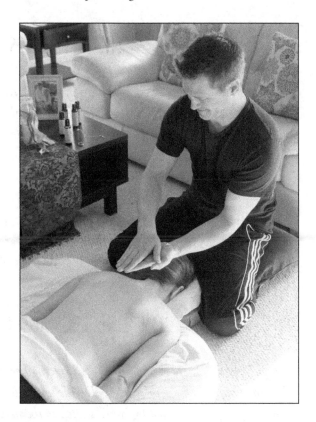

Warm the oil by rubbing the oil in the palms of your hands first before touching her back.
(Jaymie Garner)

❖ **Get slow:** Slow down. Couple's massage, unlike some other forms of touch, is all about taking your time.

❖ **Keep in flow:** Consistent contact with your partner's body is import-ant. Keep one hand on your partner at all times, even when reaching for more oil.

In the massage routine that I walk you through here, the giver is in the kneeling position. If you prefer to sit beside your partner, that's okay. You may even feel like changing from one position to another. That's up to you, your setting, and how your body feels. Find the position (or positions) that feels the most comfortable for you and go with it.

THE FIVE ZONES

I am starting facedown back up, to give you a leg up on the receiver's comfort. It's easier for the receiver to relax into the massage this way. If you are giving the massage, testing your skills on the back is going to help you prepare for the more vulnerable and softer parts when you flip your partner over.

I've divided the body into ten different zones—five facedown and five faceup—to make it easy for you to get around it. Remember, spend time on each of the zones, providing pleasure to your partner and giving an equal amount of time to every part. However, you are going to find some places where you may want to spend longer, and that's okay.

ZONE ONE: LEGS AND CALVES

Begin by kneeling at your partner's feet, facing her soles. Don't forget to use a pillow under your buttocks for your comfort. Decide which leg to work on first; once you finish the massage steps on the first leg, you'll switch to the next leg and repeat these steps.

Forget about the feet! I'll cover them in chapter 7. If you like, as a nice way to say hello, greet the feet with your hands, warming them up.

Always avoid putting pressure on the back of the knee. Do not massage over varicose veins. Avoid anything that appears swollen or is sore to the touch. Hairy legs require globs of oil, so be sure to use extra oil on the hair before you glide along her sore calf muscles.

CALVES

Legs do a lot of work and can really get tired and sore. The calves, in particular, love a good massage. However, the calves can be very tender when touched with pressure, so go easy.

1. Use the roll-it stroke up and down the entire leg 10 to 15 times, leaning forward and into the stroke to warm up the leg and increase circulation. Once the leg is warm and you feel comfortable doing the stroke, limit the stroke to the calf—from the ankle up to the back of the knee—at least a couple of times.

2. Move to the side of the leg that you are massaging and begin performing the knead-it stroke up the calf. Now might be a good time to quietly check in with your partner to see whether she would like you to apply more or less pressure.

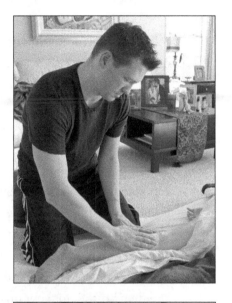

Work your way up the entire back of the leg using the roll-it stroke.
(Jaymie Garner)

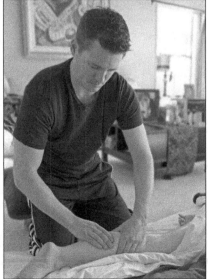

Knead-it stroke on the calf
(Jaymie Garner)

UPPER LEG/BACK OF THIGH

The upper leg is the home of the hamstring—the thick, strong, and usually very tight muscle that is sensitive to touch. If you sit long hours, this can become very contracted, causing tightness and attracting injury.

3.   Still kneeling to the side of the leg, start with the roll-it stroke up and down the upper leg. Do this 10 to 15 times.

4.   Next use knead it, again up and down the length of the leg. Try following a figure-8 pattern as you go. Repeat once or twice.

5.   Switch back to roll it, this time focusing on the inner thigh. Reaching across her leg, pull the inner thigh toward you. Remember to reach and pull with your entire body, not just your hands. Move as high up the inner thigh as you feel comfortable.

6.   Finish the upper leg with tap it and then brush it for your finale.

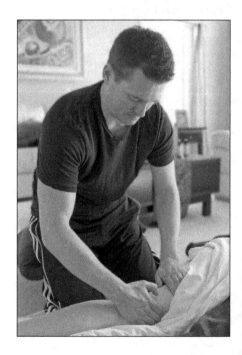

Knead-it stroke on the back of the thigh
(Jaymie Garner)

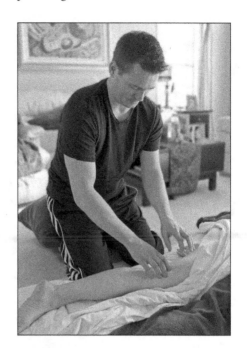

Tap-it stroke on the entire back of the thigh
(Jaymie Garner)

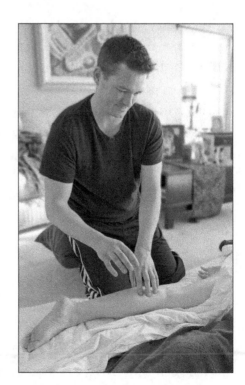

Tap-it stroke on the entire back of the calf
(Jaymie Garner)

Now switch sides and repeat steps 1 through 6 on the other leg. Be sure to remain in body contact with your partner when you are moving around her body.

> *If you are in the middle of giving your couple's massage and are working from the bottom up, facedown, your partner's arms may begin to lose sensation. When her hands are resting above her head, on the floor, or on any other platform, they will eventually go numb. If the arms are down by her side, she has a better chance of maintaining circulation in the arms. Give her a pillow so that she doesn't have to use her arms to support her head.*

ZONE TWO: BUTTOCKS

The gluteus maximus, a.k.a. butt, is one of the thickest muscles of the body, if not the thickest. Usually this is tight, especially if you are athletic. Sitting for hours at a computer or behind the wheel doesn't help either, as it results in poor circulation.

To begin massaging the buttocks, kneel at the side of her body, on the same side as the cheek you're about to touch, with your knees facing her body perpendicular to it. To change cheeks, change sides.

1. Use a light roll-it stroke to spread the oil around, or repeat the whole leg roll it from the ankle to the fleshy mounds. Do this 3 to 10 times.

2. Start at the top of the fleshy part of the buttocks and use the knead-it stroke, alternating between using your fingers and your knuckles.

Move to the other side and repeat steps 1 and 2 on the other cheek.

ZONE THREE: BACK

The back is your basic platform for all other body parts—those thick, dense muscles support the whole body, making this a perfect place to do your deep plunge into touch. If you can learn to do all of the back strokes, you can become a master of the whole body.

Although you shouldn't massage the spine itself, the muscles next to the spinal column (about one inch from the center line) produce some of the most intense sensations in the whole body when touched. The shoulders also love to be touched, as they carry a huge amount of tension and stress.

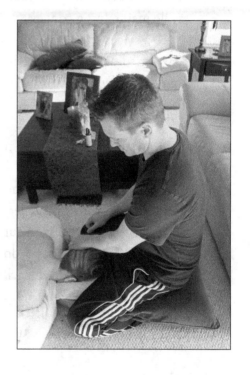

Kneel at the top of your partner's head so that you're looking down at her from her head to her toes. Your hands should be pretty warmed up by now; however, if they're not, rub them until they feel warm to you.

Brush your partner's hair to one side or clip it up before applying oil to her back so you don't get oil in her hair.
(Jaymie Garner)

---

1. Start with roll it, 3 to 10 times, with a nice long gliding movement, from the shoulders down to the waist. Then spread your hands around the hips, pulling back along the sides of her body, and finishing up at the shoulders. You may want to keep gliding in one unbroken movement, ending up around the shoulders. Try not to break contact while

you massage the back. (This may be a good time to tell her to remember to breathe, in case she's headed for outer space by now.)

2. Next, you can scoot to the side of her body and use the roll-it stroke from the side. This will give you access to her ribs, stroking across her body from one side to the other. Try some finger painting here as well.

3. Now use knead it on her sides, reaching across and working on the opposite side, just like with your roll-it stroke. Knead along the sides up into the shoulders, coming back around the other side of her body, while maintaining contact.

4. Try out some tap it along the fleshy part of the back and over those tight shoulders. Be sure to avoid tapping on the kidneys, which are located just above the waist.

5. Repeat steps 2 through 4 on the other side of the back.

6. Return to the top of her head and finish up with some energetic brush it, using your fingers. You may want to do brush it from the lower back up to the shoulders and neck area for your finale.

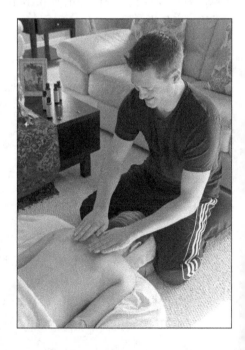

Ready for the roll-it stroke on the back
(Jaymie Garner)

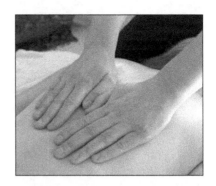

Roll-it stroke, taking care to avoid the spine
(Jaymie Garner)

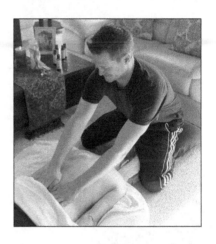

Roll-it stroke, ready to spread your hands around the hips
(Jaymie Garner)

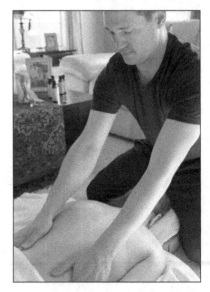

Roll-it stroke, up the side of her body
(Jaymie Garner)

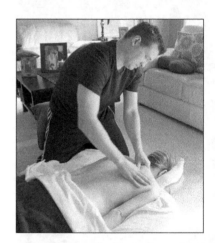

Roll-it stroke, finishing up at the shoulders
(Jaymie Garner)

Knead-it stroke on the shoulders. Make sure you're reaching across your partner's opposite side.
(Jaymie Garner)

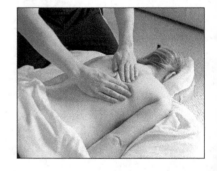

Finger painting: a variation of roll-it stroke loosens up tight muscles under the shoulder blade
(Jaymie Garner)

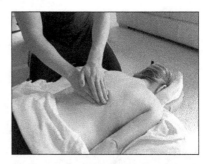

Finger painting on the muscles at either side of the spine feels really good.
(Jaymie Garner)

Tap-it stroke feels great after all the knead-it and roll-it strokes.
(Jaymie Garner)

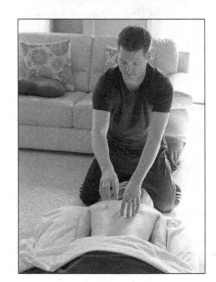

Brush it ends the back routine.
(Jaymie Garner)

ZONE FOUR: NECK

The neck supports the head, each day holding up about 10 to 15 pounds of weight. (And you thought your brain was just mush.) If you spend long hours in front of a computer and have poor back posture, your neck is going to absorb the strain. Poor sleeping positions, such as lying on your stomach with your head to the side, also contribute to neck strain.

> To avoid neck strain, encourage your partner to move her head from side to side from time to time if you don't have a face cradle. If her neck gets sore, she may need a softer surface to support her head, or roll up a towel and let her use it for head support under her forehead, elevating the whole head. Or you can invest in a U-Shaped Neck Pillow as I mentioned in chapter 3.

To begin working on the neck, remain kneeling in front of your partner's head; or if you prefer, you can also sit to the side of her neck for better angles in your reach. Again, use a pillow to support your body if you are kneeling.

1. Start with knead it. Place your fingers on the sides of the neck, starting at the base and moving up to the back of the skull. You might want to knead in small circles using your fingers or your knuckles. Don't hesitate to move from the neck to the upper shoulders.

2. Use brush it down the back of the neck (I don't recommend tap it on the neck).

ZONE FIVE: HEAD

Like the neck, the bony head can be a high-tension area. Also like the neck, the head is one of the more sensuous parts of the body.

74

Remain kneeling at the top of your partner's head.

1. Move the scalp—not the hair—with your fingers in a circular motion based on the knead-it stroke.

2. Play with the hair, letting it sift and roll through the fingers. Pretend to wash her hair, using a scrubbing motion. Go as long as you like, but be sure to do at least a full minute. Releasing tension in the scalp goes a long way to complete relaxation.

At the back of the head you will notice a little rim, known as the occipital ridge—you can feel where your fingers actually sink in. Putting your hands there is comforting and relieves tension. Ask your partner for feedback when you very gently push on it. No nails, now. Go easy and hold your pressure on the points for 30 seconds to a full minute.

If your partner is in facedown mode, it's going to be difficult to reach the full scalp. Hang on until it's time to do the pancake flip and get it then.

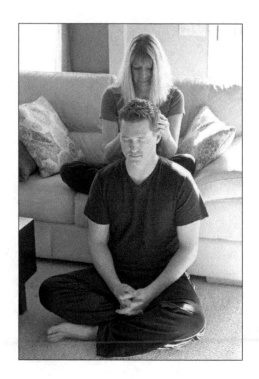

The scalp massage can also be done on a separate occasion while you're relaxing on the sofa. This can be a great 20-minute massage session before bed after a long workday. (Jaymie Garner)

75

YOUR TOUCH NOTES

❖ Before you begin your massage, run through our pre-massage checklist.

❖ How you approach the five facedown zones is a key to your success as a giver.

❖ Each of the five facedown zones has unique characteristics that must be considered before you touch them.

CHAPTER 7:
Back Down, Faceup: Massage Round #2

WHAT YOU'LL LEARN

❖ The five zones of the body faceup
❖ Massaging the five zones
❖ Wrapping up or switching roles

Once you've finished massaging the first five zones, it's time to turn your partner over and start all over again from the other side. Softly whisper something like, "Honey, it's time to turn you over now." He may be asleep, so be careful not to startle him.

Once you have turned him over and have gently positioned the legs and arms, align his body in a straight line. Gently pull his neck to straighten it, making sure the chin is dropped forward to lengthen the neck. If your partner has long hair, be sure to move those locks out of the way from under his back. Put a pillow or rolled-up towel under his knees for support. This will help to keep his body in alignment for your touch.

Just as with the back side of the body, you should focus on your partner's comfort. Check in to make sure he's warm enough but not too warm. Keep those oils at a nice warm temperature. Check how much time you have left on the CD or playlist and change it if necessary. Also make sure that you are comfortable, using that pillow under your knees. If you feel the urge, go to the bathroom now (and have your partner do the same if he needs to), before you begin round two.

THE FIVE ZONES, BACKSIDE DOWN

This side of the body is more vulnerable to injury—things are softer, more easily squished, and even more delicate, like the shins, the breasts, the genitals, and the clavicle. Try to avoid putting too much pressure on those more sensitive parts. Your massage mate is going to love it if you spend equal time on every delicious zone on this side of the body.

ZONE SIX: FEET AND LEGS

Few things in life feel better than a good old-fashioned foot massage.

FEET

Feet are bony, tender, and ticklish. Because we shove them into shoes all day, they tend to be tight and tender and suffer from a lack of circulation. Nonetheless, feet are notorious for being highly sensitive as a pleasure zone and are prone to tickling sensations, especially in between the little piggies.

To begin your faceup massage, kneel at the bottom of the feet, facing the soles.

1. Begin by rotating the ankle joint by moving the foot from side to side, first one way and then the other. Do this a few times.

2. Grasp the top of the foot, near the toes, and use roll it to open up the soles of the feet. You can use either your fingers or your knuckles; using the knuckles allows you to apply more pressure, which should be firm but not too deep, especially if your partner is ticklish on his feet. Do this 10 to 15 times.

3. Switch to the knead-it stroke, moving from the arch of the foot to the toes. Move slowly, like a little snail inching up the shaft of a plant.

4. Moving on to the toes, gently rotate each one, first one way, then the other.

5. Then use roll it to rub up and down each toe a few times.

6. Knead the toes as you did with the soles.

7. Finish off the toes and foot with the brush-it stroke on the top and underside of the foot.

Repeat steps 1 through 7 on the other foot.

While stroking the feet, you may want to place your partner's feet on your knees (if you are in the kneeling position). This gives you better leverage to touch his foot, and he can relax his leg.

Special foot massage balms and oils can enhance your massage. If you use a peppermint, eucalyptus, or wintergreen scented foot oil, be sure that you wash your hands thoroughly before touching the face or the eyes. Alternatively you may want to end with their foot massage and wash your hands immediately.

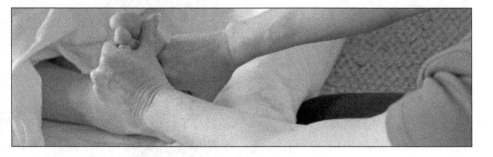

Roll-it stroke on the sole of the foot
(Jaymie Garner)

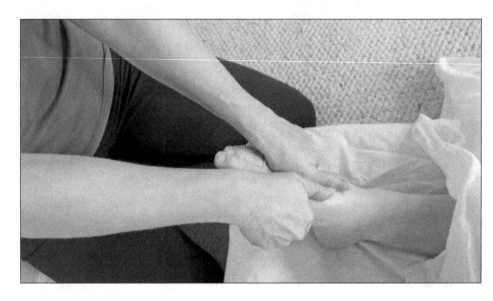

Sitting at the feet of your partner, spread the sole of the foot.
(Jaymie Garner)

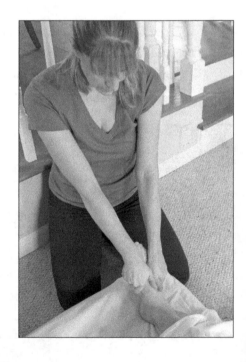

Work your way through the sole of the foot, spreading the foot as you do so.
(Jaymie Garner)

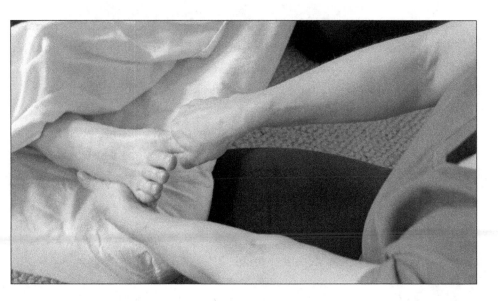

Gently rotate each toe.
(Jaymie Garner)

LEGS

A lot of tension gets stored in the upper leg, which has some of the body's longest muscles. And, of course, the inner thigh is a highly erogenous zone.

To begin massaging the legs, kneel to the side of the leg you wish to touch first. To give you more leverage so that you can push more deeply, elevate yourself from your kneeling position, leaning up and over his legs. When you are working on the thighs, remove the pillow under his knees to gain better access.

8. Start with roll it, stroking up and down the entire leg several times. Make sure you get to touch all the way up to the hips, the outer and inner thigh, and down to the ankle. Don't miss any of the leg—it's going to feel really good.

9. Focusing on the lower leg, do a few rounds of knead it. Work from the ankle all the way up to just below the knee.

10. From your same position, knead the thigh. Try following a figure-8 pattern over the entire thigh—both the inner and outer portions. If your partner's muscles are particularly tight, you can use a variation on the knead-it stroke with your knuckles.

11. Next use roll it on the inner thigh. Use long, slow strokes beginning at the inside of the knee. This is one of the most flowing strokes on the body—really lean into it and try to create a gliding sensation. If you have time or are in the mood, you can also put some frosting on the cake and do some brush-it strokes for a while.

Switch legs and repeat steps 8 through 11.

Avoid putting any weight on the knees. Light touches only on those bony protrusions.

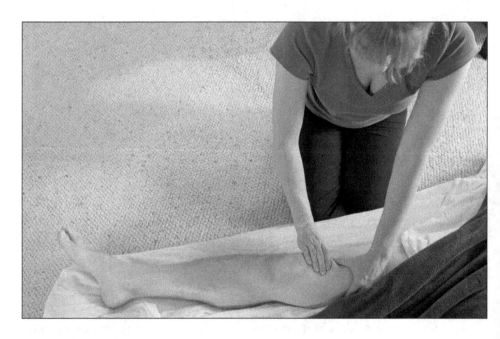

Knead it on the thigh
(Jaymie Garner)

ZONE SEVEN: STOMACH

This soft tissue area contains a lot of organs, so go lightly here. Rubbing the stomach can alleviate constipation and ease symptoms of premenstrual syndrome (PMS). This part of your body can be erogenous, especially the lower abdomen.

Start on the right side of your partner's body, kneeling to the right side of the ribs.

1. Start with roll it, stroking in a clockwise direction beginning at the navel, circling out, going up to the diaphragm, and ending at the hips. Do this around 10 times, very slowly and applying light pressure. This will release the digestive tract by going in the same, clockwise direction, helping to unblock gas, congestion, or constipation.

2. Next lift yourself up and lean over the top of his body so that you can gently knead the opposite flank or ribs.

3. Then do a roll it across his body, reaching underneath his ribs, and delicately scooping the flesh with your hands like sifting sand for shells. For added pleasure, you can even do roll it on the lower back when you do your scooping.

Repeat steps 1 through 3 from the left side of the body.

Be careful not to lean on your partner's ribs! Never adjust your posture by placing your full body weight on the bones of the chest.

If your partner's lower back hurts, this can be a good time to draw his knees up and put his feet flat on the massage surface for a few moments. It's a great way to create some relief on the back of the spine.

ZONE EIGHT: CHEST

The chest can be very sensitive to pressure, so take it easy here.

Begin by kneeling at the top of his head.

1. Start with roll it from the shoulders to the stomach, pulling your hands around the sides of the ribs, and back up to the top. You can add a rocking motion while you pull back up. Repeat 10 to 15 times.

2. Touch around the breasts in circular motions, opening the web of your own hands and letting the natural contours of the breast tissue fall around your hands.

3. Next, do some tap it on the chest, which can feel both awakening and relaxing.

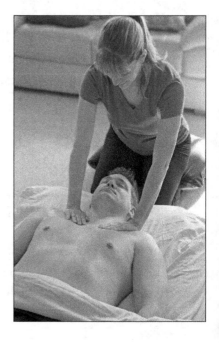

If your guy has a hairy chest or stomach, make sure that you oil the hair—that's right, the hair, not the skin. Also, watch out for the breast-bone here, especially if you are doing any tapping on the chest. The clavi-cle, or collarbone, is a delicate bone, which doesn't usually respond posi-tively to pounding or pressure of any kind. Go easy if you massage it.

Roll-it stroke on entire chest area, starting at the shoulders (Jaymie Garner)

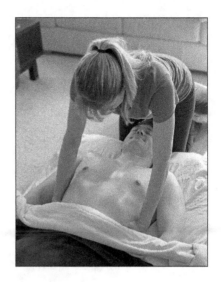

Roll-it stroke, pulling around the sides of the ribs
(Jaymie Garner)

ZONE NINE: ARMS AND HANDS

Feel free to massage the arms and hands before you massage the chest. The order doesn't matter.

ARMS

If your massage mate beefs up those biceps and triceps at the gym, a relaxing arm massage will have them sighing with pleasure. Even if your partner doesn't work out, arm massages can be surprisingly delightful.

Make sure that your partner's arms are at his sides, and kneel on the side of his body.

1. Start with a nice long roll-it stroke, from the wrist all the way up to the neck. Repeat the stroke several times.

2. Follow up with knead it, up and down the arm, once or twice.

3. Now focus on the shoulders. With one hand grasping his wrist, hold up his arm; with your other arm knead his shoulders.

4. Finish off the arms with another round of roll it, throwing in a brush down the entire length.

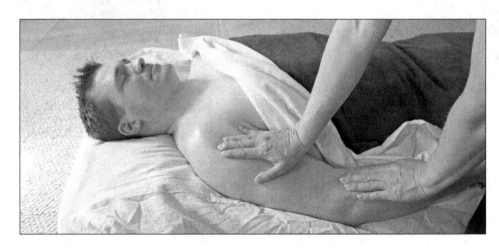

Roll-it stroke on the arms, starting at the hands up to the shoulders and back down
(Jaymie Garner)

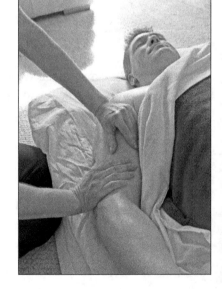

Knead-it stroke on the biceps
(Jaymie Garner)

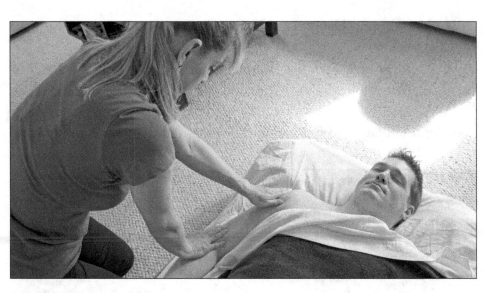

End the arm routine with brush it
(Jaymie Garner)

HANDS

Your hands tell a story about who you are and what you do, whether you're a brain surgeon, engine mechanic, painter, or sculptor. Like the hand, the palm is a secret map of who you are.

Remain at your partner's side to massage his hands:

5. Grasp both sides of your partner's hand with both of your hands and gently pull down it, massaging the palm with your fingers.

6. Next, turn the palm hand-up (not too forcefully) and hook your fingers in between his fingers to open up the palm. This should feel very relaxing to your partner's hand. Use the knead-it stroke on his palm with your thumb while your fingers remain interlocked. Before you leave this position, rotate the wrist a few times.

7. Now turn the hand over and knead the top of the hand.

8. Finally, just as with the toes, rotate each finger one at a time. Then gently use roll it on each finger, pulling the finger toward you.

Switch to the arm and hand on the other side and repeat steps 1 through 8.

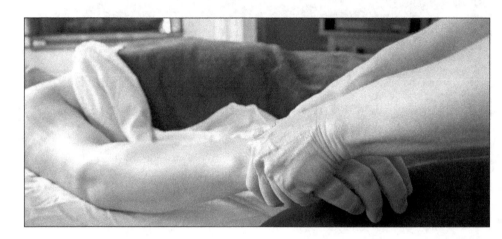

Grasp your partner's hand with both of your hands to begin the hand massage.
(Jaymie Garner)

Turn the palm hand up.
(Jaymie Garner)

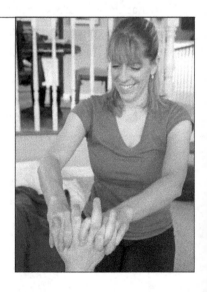

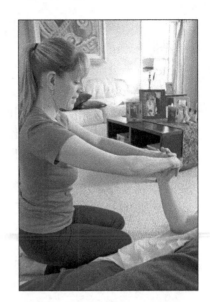

Spread the palm and knead it.
(Jaymie Garner)

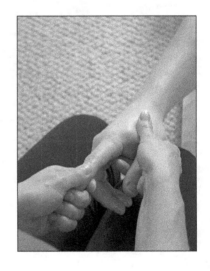

Rotate each finger and roll it on each digit.
(Jaymie Garner)

ZONE TEN: NECK, FACE, AND HEAD

When you get to the neck, face, and head, you'll probably want to change oils, using those that I recommend for the face (see chapter 3), or stop using oils altogether. If your partner has long hair, be extra careful to move it out of harm's way.

Kneel or sit at the top of your partner's head. If you're sitting, you can sit cross-legged on a firm pillow such as a meditation pillow. You can also sit straddling the head, with your legs spread down by his shoulders.

Sit at your partner's head to begin the head massage. (Jaymie Garner)

Some of my clients love scalp massage. In fact, they will ask me to spend up to 30 minutes on the scalp alone. A scalp massage can be done all by itself if you don't have time for a whole body routine.

Make sure that your partner doesn't mind using oil on his or her hair. If he or she does, tie it up in a barrette, a bandana, or a small towel. You can even place a towel on top of the head and touch the towel rather than the hair.

1. Begin at the top of the shoulders and knead the shoulders in a circular motion, working from the shoulder to the back on the neck.

2. Gently cradle the back of your partner's head and turn it to the side. Use a variation of the knead-it stroke with your fist, stroking down the side of the neck to the shoulder while the head rests in your other hand. Turn the head in the other direction and repeat.

3. Bring the head to the center and knead the back of the neck up to the occipital ridge.

4. Start massaging the temples—the area to the side of the eyes—with a gentle stroke, making circular motions the size of a small coin. Go in one direction, then reverse it.

5. Continue the circular strokes on the cheeks, forehead, and jaw.

6. Brush the chin, cheeks, jaw, and forehead to relax him further.

7. If you want, you can now repeat the scalp massage from chapter 6, focusing on areas that you couldn't reach when your partner was face-down. Otherwise, skip to step 8.

8. Finish up with a little massaging on the ears, rubbing the earlobe between your thumb and the index finger. Remember, this is a very sensitive body part, and one that can affect your health and healing.

Take special care with the eyes. Never push on the eyes. And never let oil get near the opening to the eyes—even a little bit of oil can cause serious problems.

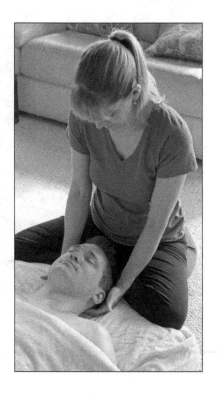

Knead it on the back of the neck and occipital ridge
(Jaymie Garner)

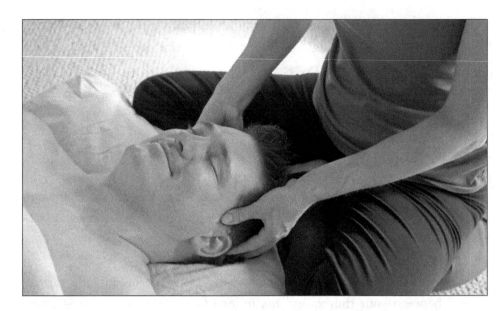

Scalp and temple massage will turn him into putty.

(Jaymie Garner)

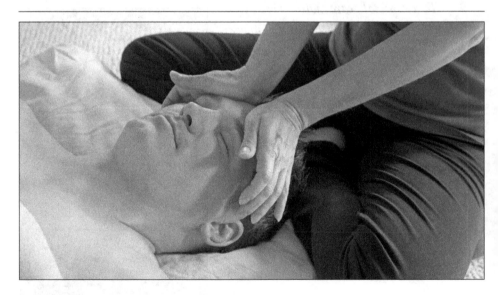

Massage the forehead by using a variation of roll it using your palms.

(Jaymie Garner)

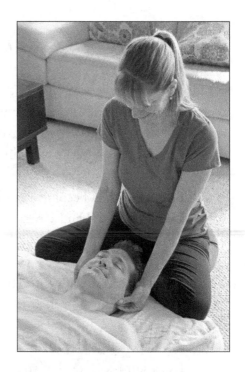

Rub each earlobe by using roll it.
(Jaymie Garner)

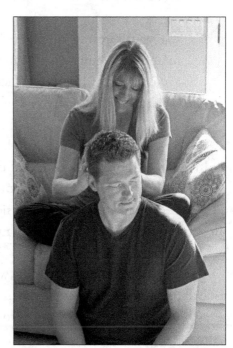

Your partner will also enjoy a scalp massage if you're short on time and don't have time to get out all your massage props.
(Jaymie Garner)

MIX IT UP

Once you have taken the time to try out the many different ways and places to do your roll it, knead it, tap it, and brush it, you may want to get a little more fancy with your touch style. I've already described some of these styles, without naming them, in the preceding steps:

❖ Roll it can also become a stroke called "Sun and Moon," which uses alternating full-hand circles in a clockwise direction. I described this stroke on the stomach.

❖ Knead it can morph into stripping, a stroke which uses the thumb and index finger to inch like a snail up a part of the body, such as the calf.

❖ Use a soft fist instead of your fingers to do tap it.

❖ Use your forearms or elbows instead of your hands, which allows you to apply more pressure. Minimize oil with your forearm and elbow to avoid slipping. If your partner wants even more pressure, cut out the oil altogether so that you don't slide.

You can integrate all of these strokes once you gain mastery over the basics. Invent strokes of your own and do your own digital creating. The sky's the limit, really, on how clever you can get using the four basic strokes and taking them to a new dimension. Even just the speed of touch, the pressure you use, and the pattern and direction of your hands can make a big difference.

You and your partner may even want to make up special names for your touching styles. Use names of dance steps, for example, like a quick fox-trot using a syncopated movement, a slow waltz to go slowly with a glide, or a mambo. Such shared language will heighten the experience.

WRAP IT UP

If you agreed that you were both going to give each other a massage, it's now time to switch roles. Before doing so, however, it's probably a good idea to take a brief break, so you each have a chance to reground yourself and prepare for the next stage.

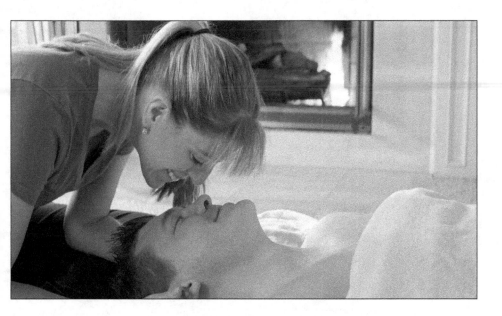

If he looks like he doesn't want to move, you may want to let him bask in the massage glow. (Jaymie Garner)

YOUR TOUCH NOTES

❖ Take a break before moving on to the other side of the body.
❖ Each faceup zone has its own special characteristics.
❖ Use special oils or avoid using them altogether when massaging the face.
❖ After giving a couple's massage, you may need a break before switching roles and beginning again.

CHAPTER 8:
Special Situations

WHAT YOU'LL LEARN

❖ Finding relief during pregnancy and after childbirth
❖ The art of baby massage
❖ Recovering from physical illness
❖ Quelling the symptoms of menopause
❖ Aging and the need for touch
❖ Giving yourself a massage

You already know that massage makes you feel great, and humans have known about the healing powers of touch for thousands of years. It makes sense, then, that massage can be used to get us through difficult physical or emotional times. This chapter will highlight some of the real benefits from a couple's massage during those more trying times in your life. Whether it's the birth of a new child, becoming menopausal, or recovering from illness, you can use couple's massage to help you cope with and even conquer what ails you.

Your partner can be your best ally if you are suffering from any of the conditions I am about to discuss. Or you can be the caregiver, using the knowledge gained in this book to help those around you feel better.

HAVING OUR BABY

Pregnancy is physically and emotionally straining for a pregnant woman. Not only is she carrying around the weight of her developing fetus, but she's also gaining weight on other parts of her body, and probably feeling drained. Being pregnant is not a sickness; however, it takes a lot of energy to sustain a woman during the nine months of gestation. With all of the hormonal shifting and body changes, it can be a stressful ride for mom-to-be. She needs nurturing fingers on her flesh.

An interesting study by the Touch Research Institute found that fathers who learned to massage and relax their pregnant wives had lower anxiety and improved marital adjustment. [Victoria Latifses, Debra Bendell Estroff, Tiffany Field, Joseph P. Bush, "Fathers massaging and relaxing their pregnant wives lowered anxiety and facilitated marital adjustment," *Journal of Bodywork and Movement Therapies* 9 (2005): 277–82, doi:http://dx.doi.org/10.1016/j.jbmt.2005.02.004. Full text available at http://spamovil.com/wp-content/uploads/2011/05/Fathers-massaging-and-relaxing-their-pregnant-wives-lowered-1.pdf]

I've already told you that couple's massage can relieve tension, stress, fatigue, and pain—all of which pregnant women usually experience. Many women who are pregnant also suffer from lower back pain from the added weight they're carrying around. Plus, they experience breast swelling, which often provokes neck, shoulder, and upper backaches.

In addition, massage can help reduce morning sickness and can even help the growing fetus: Toxins get routed through the placenta to the developing fetus, but a good rub-a-dub-dubbing can help to drain the mother's lymphatic system and reduce the chances of birth defects caused by harmful toxins. Even self-massage is a helpful relief from the aches and strains of pregnancy.

Follow your typical massage routine or the one described in chapters 6 and 7. However, instead of lying facedown, have mom-to-be lie on her side and support her belly with pillows.

Reread chapters 6 and 7 to choose what moves she feels will alleviate some of her distress. Ask her to tell you what she needs, where it hurts, and what feels good. This is no different from any other couple's massage. Mommy-to-be is going to love you for anything you can do to make her body feel more rested, comforted, less tense, and soothed.

> *I do not recommend massaging the protruding region of a pregnant woman's stomach and uterus.*
>
> *For specific strokes on a pregnant woman, use roll it down the spine, knead it on the shoulders and neck, roll it on the legs, and knead it on the thighs, hips, and buttocks. You can add a scalp massage with roll it on the temples, and for the feet and hands, use roll it and knead it.*

Any carrier oil is suitable for pregnancy, and so are rose, geranium, lavender, and chamomile essential oils. Use some or all of these in equal proportions, for a total of 30 drops in 2 tablespoons of carrier oil.

POSTPARTUM MASSAGE

Couple's massage is also a perfect antidote for those postpartum woes, such as depression, general body pain and exhaustion from just having popped a kiddo out of the body, and those common demons of constipation and hemorrhoids. The bottom line is that she's going to feel more rested and experience less tension and better energy flow and circulation if you use couple's massage.

Be sensitive. *Don't* dig your fingers into those delicate or very sore body parts. Be careful, too, that if she had a C-section, her obstetrician has approved her receiving a massage.

DON'T FORGET THE BABY!

The word is now out on massage on a baby—the crying and diapered kind, not your girlfriend "the babe." Recent research shows that babies who are massaged by their moms go into sync with their mothers' sleep patterns, thanks to the release of the hormone oxytocin. This natural wonder chemical helps to create bonding during breast-feeding and helps to propel the infant into this new sync-up with its mother. That's enough reason to rub your newborn while you're catching up on the morning news, isn't it?

Put your baby down on a soft surface, such as your bed or the crib. Begin massaging the baby's head and face, so that you can maintain eye contact. Make sure the room is warm enough and minimize noise distractions, just as you'd like to have it if you were getting a massage.

If you decide to oil up your little one, use a carrier oil such as almond oil. Place your fingertips on thumbs on areas too small for your whole hand. Keep all of your strokes slow and smooth, and watch for baby's response to your touch. Baby will let you know if he likes it or not, by smiling, cooing, writhing, or jumping for joy.

Roll it in circles on the scalp, working over the whole head. Go up and down the arms and legs, rotate those tiny fingers (softly and gently now), and take a gander at using the "Sun and Moon" stroke I described in chapter 7 on that fat little belly. Using roll it up and down the back is always soothing and will make you feel really good, too, by inhaling that wonderful scent that's oh-so baby!

A little rub-a-dubbing on your infant (clothed or not) may even put him to sleep. Now there's something every parent needs!

If you're looking for an additional guide to massaging your baby with specific techniques, my dear friend Dr. Elaine Fogel Schneider is the author of *Massaging Your Baby: The Joy of Touch Time.*

WHEN CHICKEN SOUP IS NOT ENOUGH

Chicken soup may help you feel better if you're sick, but if that's not your style, think about the benefits of touch. If you or your massage partner have just undergone surgery or are ill and in recovery, touch is essential. Of course, whether your honey just ran a marathon, was in a car accident, just had her bunions removed, or has the flu, she has to be handled with plenty of TLC—emphasis on the *care.*

How you touch someone who is sick or recovering is going to be determined by what happened to her or his body during that illness, injury, or surgical procedure. However, careful is your watchword, no matter what state he or she is in.

As noted previously, touch can help to improve circulation, oxygenate the blood, and remove those dratted toxins that cause disease later on. Some people even claim that it can reduce swelling and help to break down scar tissue. I don't think that doing a gentle session of touch on your sweetie will erase any stretch marks, but the key here is to boost circulation and energy flow around the body. If you're sick or recovering from surgery, even just the knowledge that someone cares enough to take the time to touch you will help you feel better and get better faster.

> *In recovery from recent surgery, there are some recommended protocols I want to mention. Don't ever massage over sutures, wounds, or sites of intense pain. Although some experts may tell you that touching the sites of a wound, surgery, or any other invasion of the body is good for you, I recommend that you leave that up to the professionals.*

HONEY, I CAN'T SLEEP

If you are one of the millions of people who suffer from lack of sleep, or even if you're just dreaming of that trip to Paris but are trembling with fear about the horrors of jet lag, you're in luck. As noted in chapter 2, massage stimulates the release of hormones that help you catch your Zzzz's.

Sleep is an important part of the healing process, so using a tender touch on your partner's body after surgery or a long illness will not only feel good but, by helping him or her sleep, will further contribute to his or her recovery.

THE CHANGE OR THE CURSE?

If you are a woman over age 50, you've probably already reached menopause. If you're in your early 40s, the biological clock is probably still ticking,
but the batteries are running low, meaning that you're in that period called
perimenopause. For you, hot flashes are *not* nights of unabashed passion, and
days of stable moods are a fleeting memory.

> *Perimenopause—the months or years leading up to the actual onset of
> menopause, which is technically one year after your last menstrual period.*

Many women who are perimenopausal suffer from just as many of the symptoms of body upheaval as those with premenstrual syndrome (PMS). Those
symptoms include tension, aching in the groin and lower back, headaches,
depression, mood swings, bloating, and breast tenderness. You name it, it's
probably something you can blame on either PMS or perimenopause, wrong
or right. And despite all the best intentions of medicine to help you out during
these phases (yes, there are hundreds of drugs and over-the-counter remedies
now), one of the best ways to feel better is a little couple's massage.

Combating stress, fatigue, aching muscles, tired bones, a worn-out nervous
system, and lack of anything remotely like a desire to be intimate, a couple's
massage is a good way to find some relief.

UP AGAINST THE CLOCK

If 80 million Americans have their way, no one will age in the 21st century.
However, even with the billions of dollars spent on anti-aging products and
cosmetic improvements, you can't win this battle in the end. And although you
can gracefully age, as many do today, with supplements, exercise, or spa retreats
for lifelong rejuvenation, you are going to reach a point where the skin sags

and that flesh that used to point straight forward as an arousal cue now points south on your compass. As people age, they might feel tender more often, tire more easily, and walk with a slower step. (If you do maintain a healthy lifestyle with exercise, diet, and a positive mental attitude, things will not deteriorate as quickly as they could.) When you get older, you can really benefit from touch.

Seniors don't often think they have the right to touch or be touched. They may have lost their spouses or they might live in contained environments where, except for those enlightened few, the idea of an intimate union is all but forbidden.

> *Some progressive hospitals have started using massage as part of their treatment programs for patients with Alzheimer's. One study showed that massaging the neck and shoulder areas reduced symptoms such as pacing, irritability, and restlessness.*

Seniors need skin-to-skin touch as much as supple-skinned youth. Seniors often have chronic aches and pains, can be creaky and cranky, and go slowly. If you are massaging Granny or Great-Uncle Louie, you will want to go easy, slow down, and be gentle with those sore, tight places. Here are some tips for how to give massage to an elderly person, and how to maximize their comfort while they receive touch pleasure.

❖ You will need to add extra padding to the massage surface, such as a double comforter under the sheet or a foam pad under the bedding.

❖ You can always massage Gramps in a chair, having him sit facing the back and lean on it.

❖ A scalp massage or a rubbing all over the head will bring great relief.

❖ If your older friend is frail, his circulation may be poor. Use roll it up and down the back and especially on the limbs to get that blood flowing. Pay attention to the feet and hands, too.

❖ Older people may be shy about being touched. It's not necessary to remove clothing, and focusing on the hands, head, and feet may be a lovely way to create comfort, both psychological and physical.

❖ I recommend using the roll-it and knead-it strokes for maximum pleasure on your older massage mate, especially on the back and shoulders, where everyone seems to hold tension, no matter how old.

❖ If you use oils, carrier oils such as evening primrose or sesame are best for older skin types. Sesame is also good for rheumatism and arthritis. Be sure to dilute either of these oils (at around 10 percent) with a lighter carrier oil such as grape seed.

Seniors can also help others and at the same time help themselves: Older folks who hold babies and touch them not only help the babies but also get from the experience a sense of purpose and worth. Integrating couple's massage will increase your quality of life no matter how old you are!

Here's a study to prove this theory. In the study, elderly retired volunteers gave massage to infants and were compared with those receiving massage themselves. After the first and last day sessions of giving massages, the elderly retired volunteers had less anxiety and depression and lower stress hormones. Over the three-week period of the study, depression and stress neurotransmitters decreased and lifestyle and health improved. [Tiffany Field, Maria Hernandez-Reif, Olga Quintino, Saul Schanberg, Cynthia Kuhn, *Journal of Applied Gerontology* 17, no. 2 (1998): 229–39, doi:10.1177/073346489801700210.]

THE ART OF DO-IT-YOURSELF

If you don't have a regular partner or if getting touched by another human being gives you the willies, then self-massage may be your best bet. Touching yourself may seem like an odd idea, especially with all this talk about back-rubs. But let's face it, your body needs soothing touch as much as anyone's does. Without a trusted massage buddy around, doing the solo thing can be a wonderful way to relax, feel more alive, promote self-healing, and ease those achy muscles.

Self-massage might sound difficult—so how do you reach around and ooze into those tight shoulders?—but it's not really that hard. For a sufficient self-massage, allow plenty of time. Be sure to give yourself at least 15 minutes to nurture your whole body, front and back, bottom to top, with your favorite oils.

Follow the pattern I used for partner massage in chapters 6 and 7 as much as possible, starting from the feet to the head, then flip yourself over. Or use these easier-to-do-on-yourself guidelines:

❖ Lie faceup on your back, and focus on your head, scalp, face, and chest first. Use your favorite oils, just as with a partner, to create the mood you want. Of course, I am assuming that you've gussied up the place and done all the necessary steps to have an uninterrupted time at it, such as dimmed the lights, turned off your phone, set the temp control, and locked up the kids or pets.

❖ While lying faceup, continue to rub and caress yourself along the front of your torso, on the belly and abdomen. Don't forget to massage your arms and hands. Spend a good amount of time on those paws, both the palms and tops, to soothe your tension.

❖ Now sit up and pay some attention to your legs, starting at the feet and toes, working your way up. Spend a lot of time on the feet. They are probably your most overworked body part.

❖ Stand up and stretch your arms around yourself. Touch and caress what you can of your back. Draw oils or lotions around your ribs and smoosh some on your lower back where you can reach. If you bend down, you can massage your buttocks and the backs of the legs. (Right about now you'll be wishing you had practiced your stretches in yoga class a little more.)

A tennis or golf ball can be a self-massager's best friend. Lie on the ball (or balls) wherever you feel tension, strain, or stress. I guarantee that you'll feel more relaxed, calm, nurtured, and soothed after rolling around on a tennis ball for a while.

YOUR TOUCH NOTES

❖ Aches and pains associated with pregnancy can be alleviated using massage.

❖ A gentle massage can help you recover from illness and surgery.

❖ Menopausal symptoms may benefit from touch.

❖ As you age, don't stop touching.

❖ With a little practice, self-massage can feel great.

CHAPTER 9:
Location, Location, Location

WHAT YOU'LL LEARN

❖ Finding suitable places for your massage
❖ Getting your space ready
❖ Making all the necessary preparations
❖ Gathering the right materials
❖ Following certain principles to make it a success

When it comes to preparing a space for your couple's massage, the possibilities are endless. I can say this with confidence because I've been coaching couples for decades on how to bring the elements of touch into their relationships. Whether you choose a French provincial boudoir or the workout room in the basement really doesn't matter. What does matter is how you prepare the room or space, what tools and accessories you bring to the process, and how carefully you plan. This chapter is going to get you started on finding and setting up locations for your couple's massage that are going to help you move into the mood. It doesn't have to be the Taj Mahal to feel luxurious enough for a grand afternoon or evening of touch.

PICK A PLACE

Where you do your couple's massage may be just as important as what you do! Yes, that's one of the secrets to a successful journey into the pleasure and fun of touching someone else.

Don't get stuck in the rut of thinking that everything has to happen in the same place. Forget about your bed, if that's a place to crash and burn after party night, or a hideaway after too many hours at the office. Instead, get creative. Couple's massage is going to require that you find places or settings where you can lie down and get naked or close to it, so the front porch is probably out of the question. However, creating the best location may be as easy as moving some furniture.

In picking a place, the eyes don't always have it. You'll need to use all of your senses when choosing the best location. Yes, you want to make sure the space is appealing to the eyes, but you also want to make sure that it's an appropriate temperature and that there aren't any distracting noises or smells.

One woman, a lovely older client I'll call Marie, told me how her husband had set up a massage room in their house that was next to a noisy street. Just as they were getting into the relaxation of their couple's massage, booming music from a car idling outside rattled their teeth and the windows. They slammed the windows shut and laughed at how impossible it seemed at the moment to feel relaxed.

To create the best massage location, you need to not just consider the comfort of the room, but other factors such as temperature, outside disturbances, and the overall energy and ambiance the room creates.

INSIDE THE HOME

If you live in a private home in a natural location, a secluded deck might be the perfect choice. And if that deck overlooks a grand vista, all the better! Most of us, however, will have to find a serene location inside our homes or apartments.

Consider the following possibilities inside your home:

On the (sturdy, please) dining room table

On a massage table

On the floor in front of the living room window

On the couch

On the floor in front of the fireplace

The ideal temperature for a couple's massage is 72°F. Set your thermostat/ air conditioner to approximate this and you'll hit the optimal comfort zone for your body. Remember, too, that the person giving the massage will heat up faster than the person receiving it, so use the recipient as your guide for when to adjust the temperature.

Consider the following additional factors when choosing a room:

❖ **Is the room quiet and private?** Are you constantly being distracted by noises from the outside world or noises from ticking clocks and other appliances?

❖ **Is the room big enough for your partner to lie down and you to comfortably move around?** You may have to move some furniture out of the way, especially that annoying coffee table that you're always stubbing your big toe on. When it comes to massage areas, size does matter.

❖ **Is the room clean and free of odors that would conflict with the aroma created by any candles and incense you plan to use?** Make sure the room is tidy and well ventilated.

❖ **Are there any pictures or posters that interfere with the sanctuary you are creating?** If you would rather not remove them, cover them with a tapestry or veil.

If it's quiet outside and the weather is nice, try opening a window to ventilate the room. If not, then a fan or air conditioner set on the "quiet" or "silent" mode can help, as long as it doesn't create a draft.

Remember that when you are giving a couple's massage you will be warmer than the person receiving the massage. The temperature of the room needs to keep both of you comfortable. In the summer, keep a fan nearby, and in the winter, have a heater close by with extra blankets. Test the room with your wet finger in the air and adjust the temperature accordingly. And, of course, you can always make adjustments to the temperature and airflow as the massage progresses.

OUTSIDE THE HOME

You may want to get adventurous and take your couple's massage beyond your four walls. Bringing variety into any relationship stimulates excitement of all kinds. Plan ahead so you have plenty of towels, or a blanket to lie on, oils in airtight containers, and even a handy boom box or your phone with a playlist of relaxing sounds to create the right mood. Throw in your massage oils bag and pile in some mats or soft cushions if you like. I believe that the more creative you can get for where you do your couple's massage, the better.

Outside the home, you may choose to experiment with couple's massage in any of the following locations:

- ❖ At the beach on a blanket
- ❖ On an outdoor picnic table
- ❖ In the back of your truck, van, or SUV
- ❖ In the backyard under the moonlight
- ❖ On a weekend getaway at a lakeside cottage
- ❖ At the Ritz-Carlton hotel
- ❖ In a cheap hotel in Las Vegas for an escape weekend

❖ On a camping trip in an RV or tent
❖ At a friend's borrowed apartment

Although you may be brimming with enthusiasm about exploring a couple's massage out in the open, be wary of unknown settings. Some of the critters in the good old out-of-doors can be harmful or dangerous. Plants such as poison ivy, poison oak, or sumac can ruin even the loveliest foray into nature. Being prepared means knowing the dangers or safety of the space you select.

I guarantee that once you get started doing couple's massage as a regular part of your routine, you're going to invent places for massage that you couldn't imagine right now. You may find that there is one special place, such as a part of your bedroom or dining area, that you like to use more than others for couple's massage. That can become your permanent massage nook.

PUT YOUR HOUSE IN ORDER

Once you've settled on a place for your couple's massage, you might need to take some time to straighten it up—in other words, clear up your clutter. You don't want clutter to block the flow of energy or dampen your aesthetics. Nothing kills the moment like having to tend to a bleeding knee after you've tripped over a pair of smelly sneakers.

Marie Kondo, author of *The Life-Changing Magic of Tidying Up: The Japanese Art of Decluttering and Organizing*, writes that tidying is magic and it dramatically transforms your life. Kondo also writes that as a result of her method, her married clients report that they get along much better.

That's pretty powerful stuff. When you create order in your home or office, you begin to experience peace, flow, and harmony in all aspects of your life. Easy? Not. Simple? It is if you take the time to learn how to make it happen.

Try these four simple steps to eliminate clutter in the primary room where you want to do your couple's massage:

1.   **Take out the trash.** Gather up all of the stuff that you don't need and remove it from your space. You may have to take a deep breath, get out those huge green trash bags, and start hauling.

2.   **Get things clean.** Preparing your space for a couple's massage is part of the process of feeling good about it. Hire a house cleaner if you don't have time. Or set aside a couple of extra hours on your next day off to dust, vacuum, scrub the chandelier, polish the mirror, do the laundry, or whatever needs to be cleaned off and up.

3.   **Go shopping for accessories to do the job.** Get yourself some organizing containers for your stuff. If you arrange things into bins, or cute plastic boxes, wooden crates, or even metal trays, your place is going to get more organized.

4.   **Arrange things nicely.** Find a balance in what you need to have in the room and take out what isn't necessary. Let "less is more" be your guide. Minimize the things you have around you, and you are going to feel more alive, peaceful, and beautified in and by your space.

Now, take a look around you and smile. You did it.

> *Get a good book on how to de-clutter your home—**Feng Shui Your Life by Jayme Barrett** is one of my favorites—and then set aside a weekend for the task. Once you do it, make sure to keep it up, as that can be the biggest challenge. I know you can do it!*

One great way to create order in your home or office is to use the principles and practices of *Feng Shui*. For example, just having certain colors placed around your living room can brighten it up and attract the right energy to that part of the room. Feng Shui will help you to remove obstacles or objects that block the flow of *chi*, or energy, throughout your space. And if it's way over your head to even conceive of doing this type of thing on your own, then consider hiring a Feng Shui practitioner. It's not only an excellent way to ring your chimes, it's also sure to change the space you live in for the better. It can improve your whole life.

> ***Feng Shui*** *is the Asian art of placement of things in a space to create balance and harmony. This ancient form for "healing spaces" has become very popular recently and there are many books and courses teaching its principles.*

CHINESE CHECKLIST OF MASSAGE OPTIONS

Once you have had a chance to scout out a location, it's time to do a Chinese menu checklist for your massage. I want you to choose among the three types of approaches that you can use at home. They are our idea for how you can go for just the basics or add special features that give the word "luxury" new meaning.

MENU OPTION ONE: FIRST CLASS

This is your ideal. This approach will require that you spend time, money, and thought to prepare for it and to do it well. First Class requires a professional-quality massage table with a sheepskin pad. The table can also include a heating unit to create warmth under the sheets with 500-count sheets (cotton, percale, satin, or even flannel for those chilly winter nights in the hinterlands) from an expensive department store or online catalogue. In addition, take the following steps:

❖ Use heavy drapes to block light on your windows.

❖ Find a quiet location, avoiding interruptions or yucky intruding noises; maybe include a cascading waterfall in the room—or at least the sounds of one. And don't forget the tunes!

❖ Use oils and plenty of them. Be sure to reread the chapter on oils (chapter 3) to stock up on your every need. An oil warmer is a lovely way to really get luxurious.

❖ Perfect (dimmed) lighting is a must.

❖ Invest in those thick plush robes to cover you on and off the massage table.

❖ Have a Jacuzzi or hot tub nearby to soothe your aching muscles before or after the massage.

❖ Light the fireplace.

❖ Place a sheepskin rug on the floor for the person giving the massage to stand on.

❖ Stock up on aromatherapy products such as oils, body lotions, and battery-operated flameless candles, lit candles, or diffusers in the room.

❖ Place beautiful images around the room, such as beautiful goddess-head statues, O'Keeffe paintings, Klimt posters, photos of nature's wonders, your wedding photo or framed photos of the two of you in love.

❖ Grab an eye pillow filled with lavender beads.

Okay. Got the picture yet? This takes spending some bucks on things and really committing to making the setting and your props ready for action.

MENU OPTION TWO: STANDARD

This is a way to create a great couple's massage, but without having to spend the family fortune on it. Think economical. There's not much distinction between this approach and the next. It's pretty much about how much time, money, and thought you wish to invest:

❖ You can use a futon mattress or your own bed for this one.

❖ Use some of your best sheets, but ones that you don't mind getting a little greasy.

❖ Find some of the leftover candles from the holidays or scoop up some inexpensive ones from your local supermarket on sale.

❖ As always, the basics apply: music (use what you've got), lighting (turn the lights down low or off), and scents (bathe, then sprinkle your favorite cologne on for starters).

❖ I do believe, though, that you must use at least one massage oil if you are going to do this with success. Be creative and find one even at your local discount drug store that can get the job done.

Remember that old saw, "What you give you get"? The more you put into the experience, the more benefits you will derive. Don't cheat yourself.

MENU OPTION THREE: ECONOMY

Now I'm getting down to the wire for comfort, pleasure, and outcomes that you can count on. This approach will allow you to have a couple's massage that may be more interesting than watching the 11 o'clock news or a football playoff, but it's not going to be all that memorable.

❖ Try lying on a cushy carpet on the floor or a rug where you throw down one of your old sheets.

❖ Grab some pillows for support.

❖ Now oil up with some safflower oil from the cupboard, and there you go.

HANG UP YOUR "LET ME CHILL" SIGN

Doing the necessary planning and preparation for a private encounter in your own space may be a bigger challenge than you think. One of the common pitfalls when you're doing massage is interruption. Having quiet, private times and space is essential for your couple's massage to be effective. Whether you have a bevy of children, a menagerie of pets, or just a busy life, you need to create the mechanisms for keeping them at bay for just a few hours.

Creating privacy may require some creative thinking on your part. For example, if you have young children, who can you count on to watch them? You may want to reach out to relatives or other parents in a privacy dilemma similar to yours. First, show them your copy of this book. Second, offer to trade off days, in the spirit of good old-fashioned bartering. If they'll watch your little devils on your couple's massage days, you'll watch their little angels on their couple's massage days. A disclaimer: If their little angels turn out to be little devils, you may have to break down and pay for a sitter. If that doesn't work, call your own parents to pitch in. Maybe say the cat is sick and you need to give it medicine for the next two hours, rather than fess up to your goal of pleasure. The important thing is to make sure your babysitting savior is reliable, so you can relax and enjoy the couple's massage you'll be giving and receiving.

Set boundaries around your work emails, especially if you bring home your work laptop and work smartphone. Be committed to your time together and establish strict boundaries—it's too easy to send off another email and find yourself focusing on the response rather than giving your sweetheart your undivided attention.

SEVEN STEPS TO PRIVACY

I have found that there are seven basic things you can do to avoid the interruptions that can kill any joy in the couple's massage experience.

* **Make arrangements for the kids, give the dog a big bone, or feed the cat.** Send the kids packing to grandma's backyard for a couple of hours, barter with the neighbor to watch them, or schedule your massage when they are in school or at baseball practice. Plan well, but get the kids out of there. And keep the animals in their rooms or kennels, even if it breaks your heart for a split second. I mean it. Keep them away from pawing at your pleasure.

I was giving a couple's massage lesson once, and their dog decided to join us. He dragged in his bone and was happily chewing on it, but halfway through the session, they had to take the dog to another room. His chewing was breaking their concentration. Needless to say, we all laughed in the end, but that chewing was loud.

* **Shut the windows.** Keep out the distraction of the outer world. Sirens and car crashes don't make for good massage enhancers. Of course, if your home is in a wilderness area or in a quiet neighborhood, open your windows for air!

* **Turn on a fan, heater, or air conditioner to control the flow of air in your space.** You are going to need a comfortable temperature. Anything you can do to prevent discomfort is good.

* **Tell people to leave you alone.** If you have older children, guests, or roommates, hang a sign on your doorknob that signals an unmistakable "Do Not Disturb" message.

* **Turn off all that dratted equipment.** I mean it. No phones beeping or buzzing allowed. We are way too connected to our devices these

days, so stop the multitasking. Turn on, instead, pleasant background sounds. Play your favorite music to help block out any distracting sounds, such as the lawn mower in your complex or a garbage truck eating the trash that you threw out so that you could do this couple's massage in the first place!

❖ **Draw the curtains.** Close your curtains, drapes, blinds, or shades. You'd be surprised at how annoying it can be to have a ray of sunlight pierce your eyes when you're trying to give your beloved a massage. Even worse than the sun, however, would be the peering eyes of a stranger!

❖ **Try a natural sound machine.** If outside noise is really a bother, consider recordings that mimic sounds in nature, such as a waterfall or thunderstorm. Take whatever measures are necessary to make your time and space private, quiet, and serene. The unexpected interruption or distraction can ruin the couple's massage experience.

Make yourself a "Do Not Disturb" or "Let Us Chill" sign to hang on your door. Use it when you and your partner are giving one another massages.

Enjoying a couple's massage works best when you cut yourself off from the outside world. My husband gets a little nervous if he can't check the caller I.D. to see who's calling, but after our first couple's massage, he got the message. Don't destroy the mood by screening calls or leaving your phone on vibrate. Power your phone off.

PRIVACY CHECKLIST

I've included the following checklist to help you prepare the environment for your couple's massage and to avert the unwanted event or guest:

❖ Have I turned off my cell phone?

❖ Have I hung my DND or "Let Us Chill" sign on the outside doorknob?

❖ Have I made arrangements in advance for the kids?

❖ Have I tied up or scooted out the pets?

❖ Have I left word with my office or family that I am not to be interrupted at this time?

❖ Have I purchased a noise-blocking device to take care of unwanted noises?

❖ Have I selected the perfect music playlist or CD?

❖ Have I made sure that all the things that I had to take care of so far today are done, like putting enough money in the parking meter?

❖ Am I willing to let it all go, even if everything isn't done?

❖ Has my couple's massage partner done all of the above?

If you can't check off most of these items, you may want to postpone this particular couple's massage.

Don't you feel like a master of your environment now? I hope so. This can be an evolving process. You're not going to get all the supplies or enhance your room space to your ultimate liking on the first try. Focus on one couple's massage at a time. Now that you have the idea, make your massage area at home—or on the go—as fulfilling as your imagination will let you.

YOUR TOUCH NOTES

❖ Choose the best place in your home for your first couple's massage.
❖ Clean up your space, arrange the furniture, and shut down all your equipment.
❖ Send the kids and pets packing.
❖ Run through the pre-massage checklist to make sure you're ready.

CHAPTER 10:
Listen to This!

THE SIMPLE ART OF LISTENING

WHAT YOU'LL LEARN

- ❖ Sound is powerful
- ❖ Choosing the best music for your couple's massage
- ❖ Selecting words to make the best of your experience

Imagine the following sounds:

- ❖ A lawn mower outside your bedroom window
- ❖ The dishwasher clanking away in the kitchen
- ❖ Your neighbor's dog barking
- ❖ Commercials interrupting your favorite music on your music app

Now imagine these sounds:

- ❖ Birds chirping in the woods
- ❖ Your favorite musician playing
- ❖ Your partner sighing with pleasure
- ❖ Commercial-free music

As these two lists demonstrate, what you hear can have a dramatic impact on your couple's massage. Sounds can be soothing or stressful. During a couple's massage, when you are trying to relax and let yourself be one with the moment, sounds can have a particularly strong impact. How loudly you speak, move around the room, what's going on outside the house, and the kind of music that's playing can all affect you.

You or your partner might need music to set a relaxed mood, might respond negatively to outside noises such as a helicopter buzzing overhead, and might need to hear soothing words to guide you into the process.

TUNING IN: MUSIC FOR MOOD MAKING

Music is one of the most powerful tools for creating an atmosphere for your massage. Music has the ability to turn "I'm not in the mood tonight, honey," into "Let's do this, baby!"

Music can make you laugh and cry. It can bring great joy and deep sadness. And it can heighten the experience of the couple's massage. Scientists have discovered that music has the ability to activate the limbic region in the brain. The limbic region is ultimately responsible for developing your emotions and feelings, such as passion, romance, and nurturing.

MAKE A MUSIC LIST

With your partner, make a playlist of music that puts you both in the mood for relaxation, and if you're using a CD of the playlist, keep it with your massage tools. Then the next time you give each other massages, you'll be prepared. If you are stuck here because you don't like the same music, spend some time online or in your iTunes and try to find some mutually enjoyable selections.

Choose music that will complement the mood, not compete with it. Music that is rhythmic is stimulating to the body and has an uplifting effect. Music that is slow and calming to the nerves, with lilting strings and soft pianos, is better for a soothing massage. I do recommend changing your music selection from time to time as your senses become accustomed to the same tunes. Eventually, the familiar songs may no longer spark the fantasy your special moment requires.

Music also stimulates fantasy, which is why great romance movies usually have powerful soundtracks. *Titanic* is a perfect example. Although director James Cameron took home the Academy Award for this film, James Horner's soundtrack helped him win it. Imagine that movie without the glorious voice of Celine Dion crooning, "My heart will go on..." or the Celtic choirs and symphonic interludes that carry you out to sea.

Humans believe in the power of love, and love is an event discovered through the senses. Music plays an integral part in connecting you with the one you love and inspiring you during couple's massage.

> *During your couple's massage you don't want to get out of the groove by running out of tunes. Have at least one hour of music loaded on your phone, on a CD, or in your player. If you have to interrupt the moment to find the playlist or reload your CD, you may spoil the mood, as well as some great CDs with your oily hands.*
>
> *If you're using free Pandora, be prepared for the odd commercial interrupting your mood. You may want to consider a paid subscription if you plan on using Pandora on a regular basis.*
>
> *I have a paid subscription to CalmRadio.com and use their app on my iPhone. CalmRadio.com has 11 music categories to choose from.*

MASSAGE TUNES

Here are some suggestions for kinds of music that may enhance your ability to get into the experience more easily, or even intensify what you do or feel during the massage itself:

- ❖ Reggae
- ❖ New age
- ❖ Cool jazz
- ❖ Classical
- ❖ Romantic ballads
- ❖ Celtic rhythms
- ❖ Sounds of nature (dolphins, whales, wind, sea)
- ❖ Broadway show tunes
- ❖ Movie soundtracks
- ❖ Lullabies
- ❖ Gregorian chants
- ❖ Buddhist chants
- ❖ Native American flute music
- ❖ Soothing drum and bass
- ❖ World music

Make up your own list of what you already have in your collection and a "wish list" of those you want to buy.

If you're transferring your playlist to a blank CD, consider purchasing some 80-minute CDs.

If you're using your iPhone to play music, make sure your phone is set on Do Not Disturb in your settings. Consider buying a Bluetooth speaker to enhance the sound.

YOUR TOUCH NOTES

- ❖ What you hear can influence how you feel.
- ❖ Music is a powerful tool in your couple's massage.
- ❖ Make what you say during a couple's massage count.

CHAPTER 11:
Mmmm ...
Smells Good, Tastes Great

WHAT YOU'LL LEARN

- ❖ All about essential oils
- ❖ Aromatherapy and its origins
- ❖ Flowers can say it all

Ever walk by a bakery and have the aroma of warm chocolate croissants remind you of your romantic time in Paris? Or does the smell of a certain aftershave or cologne take you back to high school and the guy who got away? Imagine life without the scent of exotic perfumes, roasted coffee beans, or freshly cut grass. Perhaps more than any other sense, smell can transport you to your past just from a passing whiff. Harnessing the power of smell for your couple's massage by using carefully selected essential oils, lighting aromatic candles, or even setting up your table by the ocean's salty spray can take your experience to another level.

MAKES SCENTS TO ME

It wasn't until 1937 that French chemist René-Maurice Gattefossé coined the term "aromatherapy," although people had recognized the healing properties of aromatic plants for centuries. Aromatherapy uses essential oils (the liquid that is present in tiny droplets or sacs) from plants for the purpose of healing. An essential oil is what gives a rose its fragrance.

125

When essential oils are inhaled through the nasal passages or absorbed through the skin, they travel to the limbic region of the brain, which is responsible for memory and emotion.

Once you open yourself up to your emotions, there's no telling what can happen. Those open, warm, juicy feelings of closeness or soft, gentle vulnerabilities may be all you need to be perfectly attuned for a tender touch exchange.

As noted in chapter 3, you can purchase essential oils from your local health store and add them to your carrier oil for your couple's massage. The type of essential oil that you choose will determine the outcome: You can choose oils that are stimulating and invigorating or oils that are soothing and relaxing. The following table lists some properties of common and not-so-common essential oils.

ESSENTIAL OILS AND THEIR PROPERTIES

	Aphro-disiac	Calming	Cleansing	Sedative	Soothing	Stimulating	Warming
Cedarwood			✓			✓	
Chamomile		✓	✓		✓		
Cinnamon			✓				
Clary sage				✓			✓
Clove			✓				✓
Cypress				✓			
Eucalyptus			✓				
Frankin-cense		✓					
Jasmine	✓		✓			✓	
Lavender		✓		✓			
Orange				✓			
Patchouli	✓		✓				
Pepper-mint						✓	

Rose	✓	✓	✓		✓		
Rosemary							
Sandal-wood	✓	✓			✓	✓	
Tea tree			✓				
Winter-green						✓	✓
Ylang ylang	✓			✓	✓		

Essential oils are highly volatile, meaning that they easily evaporate. Store them in dark glass containers away from direct sunlight. They should not be used directly on the skin, as they are potent and could irritate it. Always use them blended with a carrier oil by placing 5 to 15 drops of essential oil into 1 ounce of carrier oil.

SYNERGY

Essential oils can also be blended together, which is known as synergy. One of our favorite blends for couple's massage is jasmine and ylang ylang, equal parts of each. The jasmine is stimulating and the ylang ylang is soothing and sedative. For a calming effect, lavender is always the best, in combination with orange oil. To create a stimulating result, pour equal amounts of peppermint and rosemary oils into a diffuser for burning.

If romance is your goal, then here are three special "love potions" to set the mood. For an aphrodisiac massage combo, use anything with rose or ylang ylang, especially to ignite the fires in women. Put a few drops of each in a bowl of warm water, a diffuser, or even on a candle stand for at least 20 minutes in the room before you begin your massage. Another love treat is made by placing a few drops each of jasmine, rose, sandalwood, and bergamot in a carrier oil for the massage itself. Finally, you can add 10 drops each of ylang ylang, jasmine, sandalwood, patchouli, and clary sage into your bath to enhance your readiness for romance.

If you prefer to purchase essential oils already blended in a carrier oil, I have a product line called Natural Aromatics. You can choose from five different massage oil blends. The massage oil contains grape seed oil, which will help your hands glide with ease. Depending on your mood, you can choose from five different blends of essential oils.

You can purchase them on my website here:

http://www.servethegoddess.com/goddess-oils-skincare/

WHAT'S YOUR FAVORITE?

Discuss with your partner the smells you both like and associate with relaxation. Visit your local health food store (or look in Appendix A for suggested online and mail order outlets) and pick out the scents you both like. Don't make the mistake of massaging your partner with rose oil if he would prefer a woodsy aroma like sandalwood or green fir. Consider the following scents:

❖ Musky scents, such as sandalwood, patchouli, anything woodsy, or pure musk itself

❖ Natural citrus smells, such as lemon, orange, or grapefruit

❖ Nutty odors (this is not a judgment call about your mental health), such as coconut, sesame, or almond

❖ Flowery scents, such as rose, lilac, jasmine, or perfumed blends

❖ Odorless oils, a pure carrier oil like grape seed, or a professional massage oil base

- ❖ Romance-setting oils, such as the commercial preparations sold by Kama Sutra or other brands like mine, or jasmine or ylang ylang oils

- ❖ Sporty oils, such as wintergreen, rosemary, or eucalyptus

Take a handful of coffee beans with you to the store when you're shopping for essential oils. Sniffing the beans in between sniffing the different aromas will clear the nose.

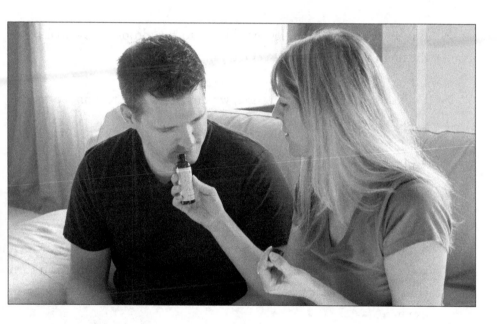

Spend some time smelling different blends of massage oils. Your partner may like something different from you.
(Jaymie Garner)

AROMATHERAPY TIPS

If you want to enhance the smell of your massage area but don't want to apply the oil to your body, you can try any of the following aromatherapy ideas:

❖ Drop 5 to 15 drops of essential oil in your bathwater, making sure it is blended into the water by swishing the water with your hand before sinking in and soaking.

❖ Purchase an aromatherapy body oil blend and add a few drops to your bathwater.
You can purchase them on my website here:
http://www.servethegoddess.com/goddess-oils-skincare/

❖ Buy aromatherapy candles or add one to two drops of essential oil to the melting wax of a non-scented candle.

❖ Drip some oil in a room diffuser, which converts oil to a fine spray and directs it around the room.

❖ Add a few drops to your final rinse when washing your clothes.

❖ Drizzle a few drops onto the towels or spray the sheets you are going to use for your couple's massage, adding six to eight drops to one ounce of purified water. You can use the same water as a mister, which you can gently spray into the air during your massage when you turn your partner over. Lavender and rose are good blends, or synergies, to use here.

❖ Add 5 to 10 drops in a small bowl of warm water and place it on a radiator, allowing the heat to release the scents.

A ROSE BY ANY OTHER NAME

The gift of flowers is a wonderfully romantic gesture. And did I mention that few things smell better than freshly cut flowers? A bouquet of blossoms in a beautiful vase will enhance your massage space by adding aroma, romance, and color.

The oldest evidence of the rose comes from legends and poetry which give us proof of the existence of the rose and its cultivation in ancient Greece.

Aphrodite, the goddess of love, was seen as the creator of the rose. In one tale Adonis, her lover, was mortally wounded by a wild boar when hunting. She hastened to his side, and from the mixture of his blood and her tears grew a superb, fragrant, blood-red rose. In another version, Adonis was more superficially wounded, and Aphrodite, while running to him, scratched herself on the thorns of a rose bush. Her blood started to flow at once, and the white flowers on the bush turned to red. Finally, there is a story which tells us of the origin of the white rose: Aphrodite was born of sea-foam, and from this foam, wherever it fell to the ground, grew white rose bushes.

There are other ways, too, in which flowers can enhance your experience. If you and your partner bathe in preparation for your couple's massage, carefully pick the petals from a rose and sprinkle them into the water to indulge in the colors and essences. Or leave a trail of petals leading to your massage area for your partner to find, symbolizing a pathway to love. Arrange an outline of a heart with petals around your favorite framed wedding photo. Shower petals on the massage sheets so that your loved one lies on the soft bed of petals. I recommend that you use dark sheets, as the rose petals can stain the sheets, especially if they get massage oil on them. Or you can brush them off once your honey has had the delicious visual image of them.

If you prefer silk rose petals, which won't stain and which you can store for future occasions, you can purchase them in all colors. I use PaperMart.com.

There's no better way to say romance than with roses and rose petals.

Ask your florist to save you a bag of rose petals (as they often pick off the petals to extend the life of the flower and would otherwise throw them away) to incorporate into your next massage experience.

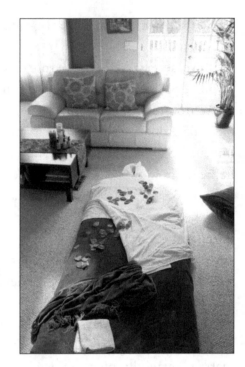

Sprinkle some rose petals on your massage platform to add a feeling of romance.
(Jaymie Garner)

YOUR TOUCH NOTES

- ❖ The sense of smell can provoke deep memories
- ❖ There are a variety of essential oils on the market, each with unique properties
- ❖ Aromatherapy can be used during a massage to achieve a desired mood

CHAPTER 12:
Communication Is Key

WHAT YOU'LL LEARN

❖ Who goes first and for how long?
❖ Making your intentions clear in the beginning
❖ Feedback—giving and receiving
❖ Communicate without the use of words

WHO'S ON FIRST?

You are about to hit the dance floor of touch, and one of you has to take the lead. It's time to choose which partner you want to be. One of you has to be the giver and the other lucky duck gets to be the receiver. If you cannot decide, then flip a coin. If that's not good enough, then draw a card and pick the highest suit. Seriously, folks, this shouldn't be difficult.

> *Think of each couple's massage as a unique journey to somewhere new. Like the geography of my home country—England, Ireland, or Wales—each hill and valley of your partner's body will be special with each visit. Think like a geographer, and you're going to find more joy each time you travel.*

WHEN, WHERE, AND HOW MANY?

If you haven't selected the best place to play lay-me-down yet, it's time to do that. Is it going to be on the dining room table, do you need to set up that new professional massage table, or are you at the beach and planning to throw down a sleeping bag? Consider rereading chapter 9, then choose a place that suits you both and take your positions.

But before you strip off those work clothes or even lock the door, take a minute to determine how much time you can devote to today's session. Do you each want a half-hour massage to start? Or is this an all-day thing? Be sure to make it fair, and even up the time allocations. It's perfectly okay if one of you chooses to receive touch today and the other gets her delight tomorrow night, for example. You can get creative here, as long as you decide beforehand how long this is going to go and who does what. Got it yet?

WHAT'S IN IT FOR ME?

Now that I have the simple stuff out of the way, it's time to take it to the next level: determining your goals for this particular massage session.

Read over the following list of reasons why you might want to receive a massage. Use it as a guide for where you'd like your upcoming session to lead. Ask your partner to do the same. Identifying your reasons for wanting a massage will help to open the lines of communication and boost intimacy, and it will also get you in the right mood. If there is a great discrepancy between your goals, it's probably time to put down the oils and grab a cup of java.

❖ You just want to have a human touch your body, anywhere, anyhow, anything. It's been months or years.

❖ You simply want to relax, forget about your worries, and just get comfortable.

❖ You have been through a rough time physically lately. Maybe you're recovering from an illness, surgery, or a baby, or medications are getting you down. You could really use some healing touch right now to soothe you and help you release some of those toxins and bad tensions.

❖ You've been overworking it in the gym and feeling a little sore. Your muscles are screaming for a good massage.

❖ You want to have your senses awakened.

❖ You want to create more intimacy in your new relationship.

❖ You're in a long-term relationship and are looking to rekindle your intimacy.

There's no need to actually get out this book and review this list every time you begin a massage, but I do encourage you to discuss your intentions with your partner each and every time you begin a massage. After all, nobody can read your mind. You may be surprised to learn that Harry has a headache or that Susie's day was too horrendous to take any more touching than the equivalent of a cup of sedative tea. Talk to your partner and you both will discover your boundaries. By the way, the more open you are about your intentions, the more likely you will be to engage in massage, because you will feel comfortable with each other.

Also remember that you can change your goals every time you decide to give one another a massage. Just because for this very session you decide you want your massage to relax you, for instance, doesn't mean that every massage puts you to sleep.

RULES OF THE ROAD: BODY TALK PRINCIPLES

You can communicate how you're feeling during a massage without actually uttering a word. I call this practice body talk, and it's a means of communication that you'll become very fluent in if you make massage a regular part of your life.

The body talks to you as you massage it. The muscles you touch talk back to you. When you are focused on your partner and really want to give her as much pleasure as possible, her body will guide your moves—it will tell you what areas are painful even if she doesn't know the source of the discomfort. Simply explore every area of her body, persuading the muscles to reveal their needs.

Body talk involves being aware of your partner during the massage. It means being sensitive to her needs and utilizing your five senses to fulfill those needs. If you are aware and in the moment, you will see your partner's muscles melting. Watch as the grimace on her face is replaced with a smile.

> *A tight muscle, like a drum skin, is hard to lift with your fingers. It is telling you that it needs a little more attention, and it will respond with gratitude when you gently knead it. A relaxed muscle can easily be lifted from the bone.*

NO MORE MONKEY-SEE, MONKEY-DO!

It's easy to play monkey-see, monkey-do. I know that you could have read a therapeutic massage cookbook—those how-to guides that offer a cookie-cutter approach to massage without acknowledging that we each have unique needs and that those needs and desires change every time we engage in massage. Are you going to fulfill your intentions simply by imitating some massage moves? A great massage, especially a couple's massage, is all about awareness. Your intention is to bring pleasure and comfort to your partner. The moment you start following a massage cookbook, you leave the flow of the moment.

The language of touch is so natural that it doesn't require an interpreter. Your thoughts and intuitive awareness can be your guides. In fact, much like a blind person can read Braille lettering, your hands can read the relaxed and tense spots of your partner's body. If you're focused on reading your partner's body, it will guide your every move.

> *Intimate body talk is like shared laughter: it brings you together. Even massaging your partner's hand can be a fulfilling event all by itself, caressing around and between the fingers and gently rubbing the soft pillow side of the palm.*

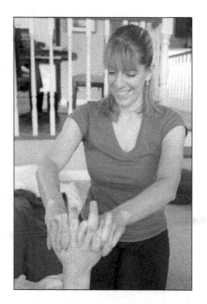

Massaging your partner's hand can be a massage session all by itself.
(Jaymie Garner)

LET YOUR FINGERS DO THE TALKING

Body talk is a two-way form of communication. Not only can you, as the giver of the massage, understand your partner's needs by "listening" to her muscles, but you can also send messages back to her through those fingers and hands of yours. The types of strokes you use, the pace of your movements, the amount of pressure you apply—these are all forms of body communication. Be sure to send the right messages.

With your hands and your thoughts, you can take your partner anywhere your heart desires. Maybe your partner has been going through some bad times and you want to reassure him that everything is going to be okay. To do this, think positive and healing thoughts as you massage him. Your reassuring touch will fill him with a sense of calm, elevate the experience of pleasure, and hasten the healing.

If during your massage a negative thought enters your mind, think to yourself "Cancel that." Otherwise your partner will pick up on that negativity.

You can transfer emotions through your hands. If you are angry, depressed, or otherwise emotionally upset, don't give someone a massage—you'll risk transferring those negative emotions to your partner. Instead, ask your partner for a rain check. Trust me, there's nothing worse than a halfhearted effort or sending negative energy to your partner's receptive body.

THE FEEDBACK LOOP OF LIKES AND DISLIKES

I encourage you to be silent and communicate through body talk as much as possible. As the giver, make sure that you aren't doing too much with your mouth—talking, that is—rather than "sensing" how it's going. There's nothing worse than, as the person getting the massage, being jolted out of a comfortable trance by your partner's loud "How am I doing so far?" Instead of checking in with your voice, use your hands as your eyes and ears. Let your hands tell you if he's flinching a muscle or relaxing into your movements. Don't keep interrupting the physical process with words. Let it all flow, better in silence than with speaking.

However, there are times when you should feel free to speak up, especially if you are the receiver and something is painful or is making you uncomfortable. Don't be afraid to tell your partner whether the oil or her hands are too cold or that she's tapping too hard. And if something feels particularly good, go ahead and moan with pleasure and a whispered "Oh … yessss." The feedback loop of likes and dislikes has to be open. That's part of the secret of a successful couple's massage.

At the beginning of your massage, gently ask your partner, "Is that enough pressure or too much?" Use your partner's response to determine how much pressure to use for the rest of the massage.

There are times, too, when the person giving the massage will need to check in. This is an opportunity to get instant feedback about what you are doing and how it's affecting your mate. He may appear to be bothered by your stroke, pressure, or movement. Gently and quietly, lean in and ask in your most in-a-sacred-temple voice, "Is that okay?" or "Too much pressure?" or "Am I hurting you?"

Use your spa voice to speak softly and just above a whisper, so no one else can hear what you're saying, as if you're in a spa.

The partner receiving the massage can whisper a quick "yes," "no," "more," "ouch," or "stop!" Or you can work out some hand signals ahead of time, such as the following:

- ❖ To show that something is painful, make a fist.
- ❖ To show that something feels good, open your palm.
- ❖ To show that something feels ticklish, jiggle your hand.
- ❖ To show that you want more pressure, put your hand on her leg with some pressure.

YOUR TOUCH NOTES

- ❖ Communication is a foundation for a couple's massage.
- ❖ Be clear about your intention before you begin.
- ❖ Giving feedback to your partner is essential.
- ❖ You can communicate without words.

CHAPTER 13:
Catch the Spirit and Be Mindful

WHAT YOU'LL LEARN

❖ **How to** honor your partner through ritual
❖ How to create a sacred space for peace and serenity
❖ Mindful techniques to keep you focused
❖ Feedback and the language of touch

HONORING RITUAL

The honoring or gratitude ritual is a wonderful ceremony for—you guessed it—honoring a loved one and showing your gratitude. It involves telling your partner why you appreciate him (or her) and that you honor his (or her) presence. If you are feeling creative, you can even write something in honor of your partner. Don't rely on trite expressions of greeting card fluff here—this is your chance to mention specific things about your partner that you appreciate. Maybe you like the way your partner has a meal ready for you after a long day at work, or the fact that he or she is always willing to listen—*really listen*—to your problems. You may honor the way your partner makes you laugh or even a little thing like the way she calls out to you when you come home. Talk about how these actions or characteristics make you feel. Get a pad of paper and start writing down some memories. If you're stuck, think back to your dating days and journey in your mind on your life together. Don't hold back. You can always edit the list before your ritual—just start writing!

I wrote down a list of things I appreciate about my husband and decided to make notes out of each item on the list. Before I knew it, I had 50 notes, so I decided to place them all in a jar with a screw-top lid. I tied a ribbon around the jar and presented it to him on his birthday. He was so thrilled by his gift that every morning for a few months he pulled out one of his notes and read it to me. This ritual made his morning and day so much sweeter.

Sit facing each other on the floor in a comfortable position wearing loose, relaxed clothing. Be natural and hold hands if you like. Close your eyes and start breathing deeply yet softly through the nose, letting your belly, ribs, and chest expand to full capacity. Then exhale all the air through your nose until your belly is pressed against your spine. Continue this breathing until you both feel a sense of calmness. Take turns honoring one another with your words. Relish the ritual as you might savor water after a long walk on a hot day. Once you've completed the ritual, you'll be focused on one another and ready to begin your massage.

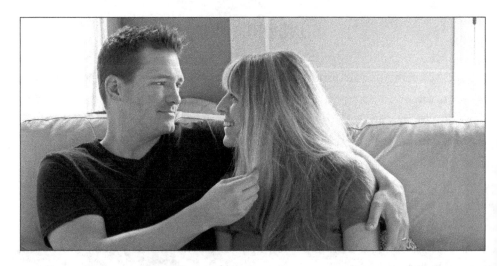

While sitting comfortably, spend some time honoring each other's presence.
(Jaymie Garner)

You may want to enhance your ritual and collect tangible items that invoke your love for each other and hold memories you both cherish. Collect a shell you found at the beach, a photo from your last vacation, your engagement or wedding photo, some fresh flowers, and an item of jewelry, and place them in front of you. You can make these a permanent fixture in your home by arranging them on a table and creating a sacred space you can return to anytime. Your sacred space is your safe haven when stress comes your way.

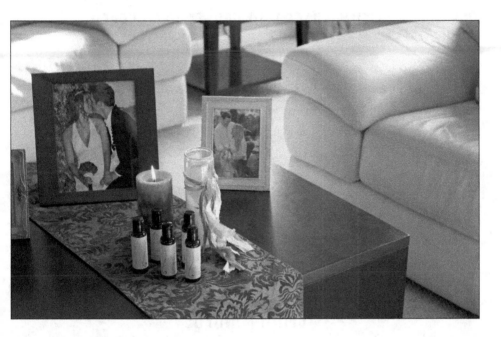

Place your wedding photo and candles on a table in your home and create a special place to visit when you need some peace.
(Jaymie Garner)

Define what "sacred" means to you. Does sacred mean uplifting, peaceful, and spiritual?

Whatever your spiritual beliefs may be, it can be calming to have a special place in your home reserved for quiet time and reflection. Find a place in your home that encourages a quiet unplugging from your day. You could use a special seat, sofa, or a small corner of a quiet room. It doesn't have to be a whole room, and it can be outside. Once you pick your special place, it will encourage you both to sit down and take a much-needed moment for yourselves.

LET THIS SPACE YOU CREATED BE SACRED

A place to keep away the negative thoughts
A place to escape the hostilities, anger, and worries of the day
A place to help keep your mind, heart, and soul cool and peaceful
A place that surrounds you with positive, loving, flowing energy
A place just for you to take care of you

> *Rituals give you the chance to celebrate the big and little things you appreciate in each other. Cherish each other through ritual, and, of course, your couple's massage.*

BEING MINDFUL

I'm not saying that to be successful with your couple's massage you must be mindful; but if you are, it certainly helps! According to *Psychology Today*, "Mindfulness is a state of active, open attention on the present. When you're mindful, you observe your thoughts and feelings from a distance, without judging them good or bad."

Instead of letting your life pass you by, mindfulness means living in the moment and awakening to experience.

In preparation for a couple's massage, I remind couples to be mindful. Why? Because we are all constantly distracted by multimedia and work demands. We multitask, and lack focus as a result. If you find yourself chatting away to your partner about your stressful day when all he wants to do is drift off, ask yourself, "Why am I talking? Why am I here? Why do I matter?"

Mindfulness increases your awareness and feelings so you can be compassionate toward your partner during your couple's massage and beyond. Mindfulness creates a space to respond to your partner in a meaningful way. It makes you pay attention and stops your reacting based on old patterns.

The Mindfulness Institute in Mill Valley, California, offers workshops and trainings, but you can start a mindful practice now by trying this 10-minute meditation.

Sit quietly and focus on your breath, taking deep, long breaths and slowly exhaling. Be with your thoughts and notice what comes up. You've probably heard the gurus saying, "Just relax," or "Release the monkey mind," but this practice can be challenging. "Meditation is easy" said no one ever. You'll be glad to know that there are other ways to meditate, such as meditating while taking a walk in nature. You can also listen to sounds, music, or make art.

You can learn to meditate on your own, following instructions in books, on YouTube, on tape, or on an app with your headphones. However, you may benefit from the support of an instructor or group to answer questions and help you to stay motivated. There's bound to be a group in your local community; just do some research.

If you have a medical condition, you may prefer a medically oriented program that incorporates meditation. Ask your physician or hospital about local groups. Insurance companies increasingly cover the cost of meditation instruction.

GET STARTED ON YOUR OWN

Some types of meditation primarily involve concentration—repeating a phrase or mantra or focusing on the sensation of breathing, allowing the ocean of thoughts that inevitably invade your brain to come and go. Meditation can be done lying down, or preferably seated, so you don't drift off and fall asleep. Concentration meditation techniques, as well as other activities such as tai chi or yoga, can bring about relaxation, which reduces the body's response to stress. I'm sure you feel the same response after a long walk in nature. Most yoga teachers in the Western world will lead you through a 45-minute asana routine to tire you out to prepare you for a 10-minute guided meditation!

Mindfulness meditation builds upon concentration practices. Here's how it works:

- ❖ **Go with the flow.** In mindfulness meditation, once you establish concentration, you observe the flow of inner thoughts, emotions, and bodily sensations without judging them as good or bad.
- ❖ **Pay attention.** You also notice external sensations such as sounds, sights, and touch that make up your moment-to-moment experience. The challenge is not to latch on to a particular idea, emotion, or sensation, or to get caught in thinking about the past or the future. Instead you watch what comes and goes in your mind, and discover which mental habits produce a feeling of well-being or suffering.
- ❖ **Stay with it.** At times, this process may not seem relaxing at all, but over time it provides a key to greater happiness and self-awareness as you become comfortable with a wider and wider range of your experiences.

PRACTICE ACCEPTANCE

Above all, mindfulness practice involves accepting whatever arises in your awareness at each moment. It involves being kind and forgiving toward yourself. Some tips to keep in mind:

- ❖ **Gently redirect.** If your mind wanders into planning, daydreaming, or criticism, notice where it has gone and gently redirect it to sensations in the present.

❖ **Try and try again.** If you miss your intended meditation session, simply start again.

By practicing accepting your experience during meditation, it becomes easier to accept whatever comes your way during the rest of your day.

Start your meditation practice at a time of day that best suits your schedule and at a time that you can stick to so it becomes a habit. Morning is probably the best time, before your household gets up and before work, or at the end of the day before bedtime. It may seem impossible to schedule at first, but consider the impact on your life of such a relatively small investment in time.

CULTIVATE MINDFULNESS INFORMALLY

In addition to formal meditation, you can also cultivate mindfulness informally by focusing your attention on your moment-to-moment sensations during everyday activities. This is done by single-tasking—doing one thing at a time and giving it your full attention. As you floss your teeth, pet the cat, or eat an apple, slow down the process and be fully present as it unfolds and involves all of your senses.

I once attended a mindfulness group, and we were asked to slowly eat and chew on a raisin for a whole 15 minutes.

EXERCISES TO TRY ON YOUR OWN

If mindfulness meditation appeals to you, going to a class or listening to a meditation tape can be a good way to start. In the meantime, here are two mindfulness exercises you can try on your own.

PRACTICING MINDFULNESS MEDITATION

This exercise teaches basic mindfulness meditation.

1. Sit on a straight-backed chair or cross-legged on the floor.
2. Focus on an aspect of your breathing, such as the sensations of air flowing into your nostrils and out of your mouth, or your belly rising and falling as you inhale and exhale. If you're not used to breathing in so deeply, close your eyes to help you focus.
3. Once you've narrowed your concentration in this way, begin to widen your focus. Become aware of sounds, sensations, and your ideas.
4. Embrace and consider each thought or sensation without judging it good or bad. If your mind starts to race, return your focus to your breathing. Then expand your awareness again.

LEARNING TO STAY IN THE PRESENT

A less formal approach to mindfulness can also help you to stay in the present and fully participate in your life. You can choose any task or moment to practice informal mindfulness, whether you are eating, showering, walking, massaging your partner, or playing with a child or grandchild. Attending to these points will help:

❖ Start by bringing your attention to the sensations in your body.
❖ Breathe in through your nose, allowing the air downward into your lower belly. Let your abdomen expand fully.
❖ Now breathe out, a long exhale through your mouth, letting out a long sigh if you wish. I like to hear the sounds and I find that it helps me release some tension.

❖ Notice the sensations of each inhalation and exhalation.
❖ Proceed with the task at hand slowly and with full deliberation.
❖ Engage your senses fully. Notice each sight, touch, and sound so that you savor every sensation.

When you notice that your mind has wandered from the task at hand, gently bring your attention back to the sensations of the moment.

WHAT IF YOUR PARTNER ISN'T BEING MINDFUL DURING YOUR COUPLE'S MASSAGE?

Don't judge. Try to be compassionate, and release your expectations. If you become more mindful, it's contagious. Trust the process and see what happens. Mindfulness opens the capacity to enjoy the moment as it deepens your awareness.

YOUR TOUCH NOTES

❖ Honoring ritual helps you cherish your partner.
❖ Creating a sacred space brings peace and calm.
❖ Being mindful and in the present moment helps you stay focused.
❖ Kind feedback helps promote better communication.

CELEBRATE THE LANGUAGE OF TOUCH

Regardless of who received and who gave the massage, it's important to give each other feedback so that you'll continue to devote this special time to each other. Be kind and open with your words. No one wants to feel criticized, and as long as you use the communication tools mentioned in chapter 12, you'll be in good shape.

Touch is vital to life, and without it, babies do not thrive. I believe the same is true of adults, so reserve time in your relationship for a couple's massage. Our lives are so busy—we talk about how stressed we are, and most of us are so touch-deprived that we often forget about the healing power of touch. Of course, it's not always possible to control the stress level in the world around us. But at home, we have the power to turn down the stress and take a deep breath. Why not take it a step further and create a sacred space of peace, connection, and healing. Honor your time now and celebrate your relationship while together you discover the language of touch.

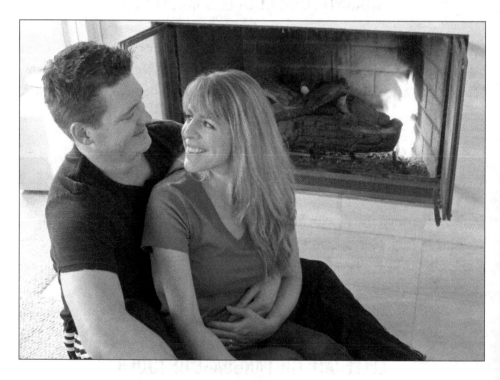

Enjoy the healing power of touch whenever you can.
(Jaymie Garner)

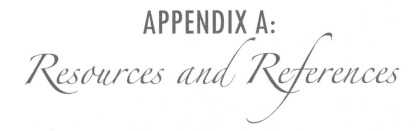

APPENDIX A:
Resources and References

- ❖ **Massage Oils**
  Natural Aromatics: Massage oil blends containing grape seed oil, which helps your hands glide with ease, available at: http://www.servethegoddess.com/goddess-oils-skincare/

- ❖ **Essential Oils**
  http://www.massagewarehouse.com/products/lotus-touch-organic-essential-oils-10ml/

- ❖ **Massage Tables and Supplies**
  www.massagewarehouse.com

- ❖ **Thai Mattress Pad**
  http://www.massagewarehouse.com/products/thai-massage-mat/

- ❖ **U-Shaped Memory Foam Face Pad**
  http://www.bedbathandbeyond.com/1/1/358919-cabeau-memory-foam-evolution-pillow-blue.html

- ❖ **Body Cushion**
  http://www.bodysupport.com/

- ❖ **Mediation Pillow—Crescent-Shaped**
  https://www.pillowcompany.com/meditation-cushions/crescent-meditation/

❖ **Music**
www.calmradio.com

❖ **Rose Petals**
http://www.papermart.com/HOME
http://www.papermart.com/bulk-silk-rose-petals/id=31359#31359

❖ **Books**
Elaine Fogel Schneider, *Massaging Your Baby: The Joy of Touch Time* (Garden City Park, NY: Square One Publishers, 2006).

Marie Kondo, Cathy Hirano, *The Life-Changing Magic of Tidying Up: The Japanese Art of Decluttering and Organizing* (Berkeley: Ten Speed Press, 2014).

Jayme Barrett, Jonn Coolidge, *Feng Shui Your Life* (New York: Sterling Pub., 2003).

KEEP IN TOUCH

I write a blog about health, wellness and rejuvenation at www.servethegoddess.com/blog/.

We can also stay connected at
Facebook: www.facebook.com/ServeTheGoddessMobileSpaServices/
Twitter: https://twitter.com/servethegoddess
Pinterest: www.pinterest.com/servethegoddess/

ATTEND ONE OF MY WEEKEND RETREATS

I also lead women's and couples' retreats three to four times a year in Southern California. If you'd like to know more, visit here:
http://www.servethegoddess.com/goddess-retreat/

APPENDIX B:
Give the Gift of Massage

Give these massage coupons to your partner, then encourage him to turn them in whenever he needs a quick pick-me-up or an entire evening of relaxation. For couples who lead busy lives, having reminders such as these helps them prioritize time for touch.

Be creative and leave these coupons in areas where you know he'll see them. One couple I coached tucked a coupon in their partner's work jacket and later in a shoe. Imagine his surprise when he finds the coupon. You'll be glad you made the effort.

MASSAGE
GIFT CERTIFICATES

You are entitled to: **20-Minute Scalp Massage**

20 minutes of healing touch to your scalp will leave you with hours of feeling relaxed.

To: _____
From: _____
Place: _____
Date: _____ **Time:** _____

You are entitled to: **30-Minute Back Massage**

30 minutes of relaxing touch to your entire back will relieve all tension of the day.

To: _____
From: _____
Place: _____
Date: _____ **Time:** _____

You are entitled to: **45-Minute Massage + Fruit Plate**

45 minutes of a rejuvenating touch to your neck, shoulders and back to help you unwind and a healthy snack.

To: _____
From: _____
Place: _____
Date: _____ **Time:** _____

You are entitled to: **60-Minute Massage + Champagne Toast**

60 minutes of re-energizing touch and a toast of champagne to celebrate us.

To: _____
From: _____
Place: _____
Date: _____ **Time:** _____

MASSAGE
GIFT CERTIFICATES

You are entitled to: **60-Minute Massage + Candles**

60 minutes of healing touch to help you feel reinvigorated and more rested.

To: _____

From: _____

Place: _____

Date: _____ **Time:** _____

You are entitled to: **90-Minute Rose Petal Massage**

90 minutes of soothing touch with aromatherapy and rose petals to help settle your senses and inspire our love to grow.

To: _____

From: _____

Place: _____

Date: _____ **Time:** _____

You are entitled to: **90-Minute Massage + Beach Time**

90 minutes of re-energizing touch to stimulate your longing for nature walks and some beach time.

To: _____

From: _____

Place: _____

Date: _____ **Time:** _____

You are entitled to: **90-Minute Massage + Breakfast**

90 minutes of restoring touch and a delicious breakfast to set you right for the day.

To: _____

From: _____

Place: _____

Date: _____ **Time:** _____

ABOUT THE AUTHOR

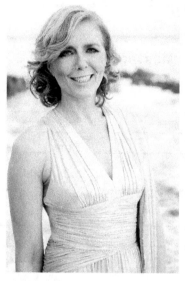

Helen Hodgson has more than 25 years' experience as a Registered Nurse and personal fitness trainer, and has been a massage therapist since 1995. Helen founded Serve The Goddess Mobile Spa Services and Retreats in 2000 after working for many prestigious salons and spas in Beverly Hills, California, and in private practice.

Helen is a licensed massage therapist in the State of California and a member of the Associated Bodywork and Massage Professionals. She is a certified trainer and the California state coordinator of the Emergency Response Massage International Team responsible for sending out massage therapists for first responders at disaster sites.

She was voted one of the best massage therapists by Allure magazine and has been featured in Massage magazine, Vibe Vixen, and Chill Out LA. Her TV and radio appearances include NBC, E Channel, Discovery Channel, MTV, and more.

She believes that through touch, couples can achieve a higher state of emotional intimacy. She has instructed countless couples on how to harness the healing power of touch with massage.

Helen also leads Women's and Couples' Weekend Retreats throughout Southern California.

She lives in Hermosa Beach, California, with her husband and cat Sephie.